P9-BXX-667

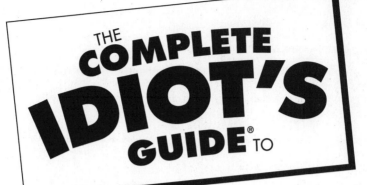

THE **COMPLETE IDIOT'S GUIDE®** TO

Vaccinations

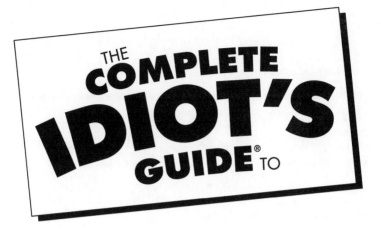

Vaccinations

*by Michael Joseph Smith, M.D., M.S.C.E.,
and Laurie Bouck*

ALPHA

A member of Penguin Group (USA) Inc.

BOCA RATON PUBLIC LIBRARY
BOCA RATON, FLORIDA

This book is dedicated to my wife and parents. Your never-ending love and support are my inspiration. —*Michael Smith*

For my husband and fellow writer, Rob, a true partner who understands a writer's life. —*Laurie Bouck*

ALPHA BOOKS

Published by the Penguin Group

Penguin Group (USA) Inc., 375 Hudson Street, New York, New York 10014, USA

Penguin Group (Canada), 90 Eglinton Avenue East, Suite 700, Toronto, Ontario M4P 2Y3, Canada (a division of Pearson Penguin Canada Inc.)

Penguin Books Ltd., 80 Strand, London WC2R 0RL, England

Penguin Ireland, 25 St. Stephen's Green, Dublin 2, Ireland (a division of Penguin Books Ltd.)

Penguin Group (Australia), 250 Camberwell Road, Camberwell, Victoria 3124, Australia (a division of Pearson Australia Group Pty. Ltd.)

Penguin Books India Pvt. Ltd., 11 Community Centre, Panchsheel Park, New Delhi—110 017, India

Penguin Group (NZ), 67 Apollo Drive, Rosedale, North Shore, Auckland 1311, New Zealand (a division of Pearson New Zealand Ltd.)

Penguin Books (South Africa) (Pty.) Ltd., 24 Sturdee Avenue, Rosebank, Johannesburg 2196, South Africa

Penguin Books Ltd., Registered Offices: 80 Strand, London WC2R 0RL, England

Copyright © 2009 by Laurie Bouck

All rights reserved. No part of this book shall be reproduced, stored in a retrieval system, or transmitted by any means, electronic, mechanical, photocopying, recording, or otherwise, without written permission from the publisher. No patent liability is assumed with respect to the use of the information contained herein. Although every precaution has been taken in the preparation of this book, the publisher and authors assume no responsibility for errors or omissions. Neither is any liability assumed for damages resulting from the use of information contained herein. For information, address Alpha Books, 800 East 96th Street, Indianapolis, IN 46240.

THE COMPLETE IDIOT'S GUIDE TO and Design are registered trademarks of Penguin Group (USA) Inc.

International Standard Book Number: 978-1-59257-930-3
Library of Congress Catalog Card Number: 2009928397

11   10   09   8   7   6   5   4   3   2   1

Interpretation of the printing code: The rightmost number of the first series of numbers is the year of the book's printing; the rightmost number of the second series of numbers is the number of the book's printing. For example, a printing code of 09-1 shows that the first printing occurred in 2009.

Printed in the United States of America

Note: This publication contains the opinions and ideas of its authors. It is intended to provide helpful and informative material on the subject matter covered. It is sold with the understanding that the authors and publisher are not engaged in rendering professional services in the book. If the reader requires personal assistance or advice, a competent professional should be consulted.

The authors and publisher specifically disclaim any responsibility for any liability, loss, or risk, personal or otherwise, which is incurred as a consequence, directly or indirectly, of the use and application of any of the contents of this book.

Most Alpha books are available at special quantity discounts for bulk purchases for sales promotions, premiums, fund-raising, or educational use. Special books, or book excerpts, can also be created to fit specific needs.

For details, write: Special Markets, Alpha Books, 375 Hudson Street, New York, NY 10014.

Publisher: *Marie Butler-Knight*
Editorial Director: *Mike Sanders*
Senior Managing Editor: *Billy Fields*
Executive Editor: *Randy Ladenheim-Gil*
Development Editor: *Susan Zingraf*
Production Editor: *Kayla Dugger*

Copy Editor: *Christine Hackerd*
Cover Designer: *Bill Thomas*
Book Designer: *Trina Wurst*
Indexer: *Angie Bess Martin*
Layout: *Ayanna Lacey*
Proofreader: *Laura Caddell*

BOCA RATON PUBLIC LIBRARY
BOCA RATON, FLORIDA

Contents at a Glance

Contents

Introduction

Everyone, it seems, has an opinion about vaccinations. A doctor, a nurse, or a parent who has seen a child suffer from a vaccine-preventable disease such as a Hib infection will probably become a strong advocate for childhood vaccinations. A parent whose child is diagnosed with autism, on the other hand, might believe that a vaccine caused the disorder. Someone else might believe that vaccines are no longer necessary because the diseases they prevent are so rare in the United States.

Information you hear in the media about vaccines sometimes confuses the issue. For example, you might hear about dangerous measles outbreaks among unvaccinated children, but also hear that childhood vaccines are dangerous because they might cause certain childhood diseases.

Without a doubt, vaccines can be a confusing topic. Part of the problem is the fact that vaccines are usually given to healthy people to prevent diseases they might never be exposed to. Medications such as antibiotics, on the other hand, are usually given to sick people to help them get better, and patients can soon tell whether the medications worked. If you are healthy when you get a vaccination and stay healthy afterward, you might not see any benefit to the vaccine you received. It's not surprising that some people have questions about vaccines.

This book tries to answer those questions. This book explains what vaccines are, how they are made, how they work, and why they are still important. You will learn what vaccines are recommended at different ages, for everyone from infants to seniors, and what vaccines special populations might need, such as chronically ill people, pregnant women, and international travelers. You will learn when you might need a tetanus booster after an injury, how some vaccines might protect us from bioterrorism, and what new vaccines you might see in the future.

This book also explains many issues that are often raised about vaccines, such as whether they can cause illnesses or injuries, why children now receive so many vaccines, and what to do if you believe you were harmed by a vaccine. It covers federal and state policies behind vaccines, such as vaccination requirements for school-age children, funding programs to make vaccines available to more people, and programs designed to safeguard the vaccine supply in the United States.

In the end, we hope that this book answers all your questions about vaccinations, and provides the information and resources you need to make the best choices for yourself, your family, and your community.

Please note that the information in this book is based on 2009 vaccination recommendations. Because these recommendations can change yearly, check with your health-care provider or the Centers for Disease Control and Prevention to find vaccination recommendations after 2009.

How This Book Is Organized

This book is divided into four sections, covering both general information on vaccines and specific recommendations for each age group.

Part 1, "Understanding Vaccines," explains where the concept of a vaccine came from, and how the first vaccine was created. We also explore how vaccines work within your complex immune system to strengthen your response to certain diseases. Lastly, you will learn how vaccines from your health-care provider are tested, regulated, and administered.

Part 2, "Standard Vaccinations for Every Age," explains what vaccines you need at every stage of life, what diseases these vaccines prevent, and why each vaccine is given at a specific age.

Part 3, "Episodic and Circumstantial Vaccinations," covers vaccinations you might need under special circumstances, such as a rabies vaccination after an animal bite or a yellow fever vaccination for international travel. This part also discusses potential vaccines being developed now, such as malaria, HIV/AIDS, and cancer vaccines.

Part 4, "Vaccination Controversies," discusses controversies surrounding vaccines, such as whether vaccines can cause disease, the use of fetal cells in creating some vaccines, when and why vaccines sometimes don't work, and what causes vaccine shortages.

Sidebars

Vaccines have influenced—and been influenced by—federal law, American and international history, and scientific advances. Throughout the book, you'll find sidebars about these and other topics to make your reading experience more enjoyable and informative. Look for these special highlights for more information:

Brain Booster

Additional information about health issues and the medical field.

Vaccinating Facts

Interesting facts and tidbits about vaccinations.

Health Advisory

Health and vaccination issues to watch out for.

def•i•ni•tion

Medical and health terms explained or clarified.

Acknowledgments

This book would not be possible without the efforts of the countless scientists, clinicians, and public health workers who have dedicated their careers to the prevention of vaccine-preventable diseases. I am especially grateful for the wisdom and guidance of Drs. Georges Peter, Penelope Dennehy, and Paul Offit. Thank you for your hard work on the behalf of children's health. —Dr. Michael Smith

I would like to thank my agent Marilyn Allen for approaching me with this book, a complex but important topic in medicine. Many thanks to my co-author, Dr. Michael Smith, for his insights into epidemiology and many fascinating discussions of the medical and social issues surrounding vaccination.

I found excellent background research online at the websites for the Centers for Disease Control and Prevention, the National Network for Immunization Information, and the Children's Hospital of Philadelphia's Vaccine Education Center. These organizations work hard to provide accurate, accessible, and timely information about vaccinations. —Laurie Bouck

Trademarks

All terms mentioned in this book that are known to be or are suspected of being trademarks or service marks have been appropriately capitalized. Alpha Books and Penguin Group (USA) Inc. cannot attest to the accuracy of this information. Use of a term in this book should not be regarded as affecting the validity of any trademark or service mark.

Part 1

Understanding Vaccines

Did you know that the first vaccine was made over 200 years ago, for a disease that was finally eradicated worldwide in the 1970s? Do you know how vaccines create immunity to a disease, and how they are developed today?

In this part, we'll explain when and how vaccination began, how vaccines work, what kinds of diseases they protect against, how vaccines are developed today, and who makes recommendations about the vaccines you might need.

1

How It All Began

In This Chapter

- ◆ How the first vaccine was created
- ◆ Why the smallpox vaccine is no longer necessary
- ◆ Concerns people had about the smallpox vaccine
- ◆ Why there are so many vaccines today

You don't hear much about smallpox outbreaks these days, thanks to English doctor Edward Jenner's work on the smallpox vaccine—the first vaccine in history—more than 200 years ago. Created in 1796 to battle this once very common and deadly disease, the vaccine was a product of folk knowledge and scientific experimentation.

Although the smallpox vaccine has since saved countless lives worldwide, many of the social and ethical concerns about vaccination that first began with this vaccine still linger. The story of smallpox provides a fascinating window into the tumultuous, experimental road to vaccine development and distribution.

Smallpox: The Speckled Monster

Smallpox outbreaks and epidemics have occurred throughout most of recorded human history. Smallpox-like rashes have been identified on Egyptian mummies, and written descriptions of a smallpox-like disease in China date back to 1122 B.C.E. The disease reached Europe around 500 to 700 C.E., and the English later nicknamed smallpox "the speckled monster."

Smallpox was typically spread like a cold or the flu, through close contact with someone infected with the virus who was coughing or sneezing. There are two types of the *variola* virus that caused smallpox: variola major, which was more common and caused more severe disease, and variola minor, which caused milder symptoms. The best-known symptom was a painful, head-to-toe rash that often left deep scars. Rashes that reached the eyes had the potential to cause blindness.

> **Vaccinating Facts**
>
> Smallpox infection caused small, blisterlike sores on the skin. In contrast, the sexually transmitted bacterial disease syphilis was sometimes called "great pox" because it caused large sores on the skin, among other symptoms.

> **def•i•ni•tion**
>
> **Variola** comes from the Latin word *varius,* meaning "spotted," or *varus,* meaning "pimple."

It was a devastating disease—up to 30 percent of people who caught smallpox died from it, and infants died at a much higher rate. In some countries in the 1700s, as many as one child in every seven died of smallpox.

Give It to Me

The only good thing about catching smallpox was that once you had it and recovered from it, you never caught it again. This discovery led scientists and others to experiment with controlled exposure to smallpox to create immunity to the disease.

Some people deliberately tried to catch a mild smallpox infection, so they could recover from it and then be protected from getting the disease in the future. What people were actually doing was performing a very primitive form of *inoculation*.

In *variolation*, a medical procedure specific to smallpox, an uninfected person was given a small amount of biological material containing the variola virus, taken from someone who had smallpox. Usually, the skin was punctured to deliver the virus to the body. Ideally, the recipient would develop a mild smallpox infection, recover, and be immune to smallpox from then on.

> ### Vaccinating Facts
>
> In one famous outbreak, in 1721, smallpox sickened almost half of Boston's population of 12,000 people.

def•i•ni•tion

Inoculation is the general term used to describe the act of giving biological material to someone to create or strengthen immunity to a disease.

Variolation is a form of inoculation used to prevent smallpox, which is caused by the variola virus.

In general, variolation succeeded in preventing smallpox, and it was practiced in Africa, Asia, and elsewhere for many centuries. While smallpox had a 30 percent death rate, the death rate from variolation was only about 3 percent. The procedure did have some problems, however, and it was not foolproof. Some variolated people still died of smallpox, or they spread smallpox to others. Some caught other diseases the variola virus donors had, such as tuberculosis—another potentially deadly disease most common in the lungs. But, while variolation had its problems, it did significantly slow the death rate of smallpox in those days.

Cowpox Power

In England in the 1700s, one particular group of people was mysteriously immune to smallpox: milkmaids. They were often celebrated for their beautiful skin, unmarked by smallpox scars. Some people believed milkmaids did not catch smallpox because they caught a milder infectious disease, called cowpox, from the cows they milked. And they were right! The virus that caused cowpox in animals caused a mild rash in humans. Unlike smallpox, however, cowpox did not cause blindness or deep scars, and it was rarely fatal. Catching the virus actually gave the milkmaids immunity to smallpox. The cowpox virus (causing cowpox in animals), the vaccinia virus (believed to be a cowpox/smallpox "hybrid" virus, and used in today's smallpox vaccine), and the variola (smallpox) virus are separate but genetically related viruses, which is how immunity to smallpox could occur from exposure to smallpox or vaccinia.

Around 1762, a milkmaid in England commented to Edward Jenner, a young surgeon's apprentice at the time, "I shall never have smallpox for I have had cowpox. I shall never have an ugly pockmarked face."

By this time, many people in England and elsewhere already believed a cowpox infection could prevent a smallpox infection. Jenner combined this knowledge, however, with the idea of variolation: what if he inoculated someone with the cowpox virus to prevent smallpox?

def•i•ni•tion

The word **vaccination** is derived from the Latin word *vacca*, meaning "cow." Originally, vaccination specifically meant inoculation with the cowpox virus to prevent smallpox. Over time, however, the meaning of the word has evolved to mean any kind of inoculation.

In 1796, Jenner inoculated a young boy with biological material he collected from a milkmaid with the cowpox virus. The boy became mildly ill with cowpox, but he felt better after 10 days. Then, two months later, Jenner inoculated the same boy with the smallpox (variola) virus, and the boy did *not* develop smallpox. Jenner called this successful cowpox inoculation *vaccination*. Hence, the cowpox inoculation to prevent smallpox became the first vaccine.

This vaccine was safer than variolation because it could not cause smallpox, and because a vaccinated person could not give smallpox to someone else (because they were vaccinated with cowpox, rather than smallpox). Yet vaccination still had some of the risks of variolation, such as giving the recipient other infectious diseases from the human cowpox donor.

In time, the English government and other European governments saw the advantages of promoting this vaccination. The procedure could protect the population against a devastating disease that had the ability to destabilize societies in large outbreaks, and the vaccination had proven safer than variolation. So by 1800, with the support of their governments, about 100,000 Europeans were vaccinated. Within a few years, President Thomas Jefferson began a vaccination campaign in America. Soon, vaccination was mandatory for citizens in many countries worldwide.

The Fall of the Monster

Thanks to vaccination, the last case of smallpox occurred in the United States in 1949. For many years, however, smallpox still persisted in other parts of the world, with rates especially high in sub-Saharan Africa, Asia, Indonesia, and Brazil.

In the years following Jenner's creation, the smallpox vaccine was refined to improve its safety. New scientific techniques, such as freeze drying the vaccine, made it easier to transport and more stable to use in the hot and humid areas of the world where smallpox persisted. In the late 1960s, the World Health Assembly—the governing organization of the World Health Organization (WHO), which is the world's primary health policy-setting body—decided to fund and promote the Intensified Global Eradication Program (IGEP) to get rid of smallpox for good. This ambitious program needed to reach over one billion people in 31 countries. The IGEP began vaccination campaigns with the goal of vaccinating 80 percent of the population in countries where smallpox still existed. IGEP surveillance teams quarantined smallpox patients in their homes or in special facilities, and then vaccinated all of the patients' household members and other close contacts in an attempt to prevent it from spreading beyond that case.

This practice was very effective. By the mid-1970s, smallpox had been eradicated everywhere in the world except in a small part of Africa. The last case of smallpox caught in the wild (i.e., caught through contact with the virus in its natural environment, not in a laboratory) occurred in Somalia in 1977. Then, in 1980, WHO declared smallpox eradicated—only a few laboratories still keep the smallpox virus for research purposes. With the world safely rid of smallpox, vaccinations were no longer required. Hence, individuals no longer receive the standard smallpox vaccination, because it is no longer necessary.

> ### Vaccinating Facts
>
> In 1977, a young hospital cook in Merka, Somalia, was the last person to catch smallpox in the wild (he survived). Two laboratory workers studying the virus in England caught smallpox the next year, and there have been no known cases of smallpox in the world since then.

The Opposition

Ever since variolation was first used in the west, it faced some opposition. Some people argued variolation would only spread smallpox, not prevent it, and it was therefore unethical to perform the procedure. Others had cultural and religious objections, thinking that variolation should not be practiced by Christians because it began in what were considered "heathen" areas of the world, like the Middle East and Africa. Others thought blocking the disease from spreading interfered with the will of God.

After Jenner developed the first vaccine, religious objections continued. Some clergymen in England called the practice ungodly, professing it was wrong to give humans an animal virus, crossing the barrier between species. In the late 1700s and early 1800s, many cartoons were published ridiculing Jenner and those he vaccinated.

In Europe and the United States, resistance from some to universal vaccination gave rise to an antivaccination movement that emerged in the 1800s. Protesters argued that mandatory vaccinations were a violation of their privacy and their bodies, dangerous due to safety or infection risks, or unnecessary due to declining rates of smallpox (even though this decline was thanks to successful vaccination programs). Many of these arguments are still used today to criticize modern vaccines. (We'll cover this topic in more detail in Part 4.)

Health Advisory _____

Contamination has been a concern throughout the history of vaccinations. A contaminated vaccine might prevent one infectious disease, but give the recipient a different disease. In the twentieth century, multiple-use vaccine containers sometimes became contaminated with bacteria after they were opened, which could sicken or even kill someone who received a vaccine from that container. To solve this problem, many vaccines are now stored in single-dose containers. Preservatives are used to prevent contamination of multiple-dose containers of vaccines.

What's Next

Although the first vaccine helped prevent smallpox epidemics, other infectious diseases still remained. Measles and diphtheria were top childhood killers in the past, and the number of polio cases spiked in the twentieth century. So, the research continued to create vaccines for these and many other diseases.

Yet, for almost 100 years following the invention of the first vaccine, no additional vaccines were developed. It was not until the late 1800s that French chemist Louis Pasteur developed the second vaccine in history: the rabies vaccine. (We'll explore the rabies disease and vaccine in detail in Chapter 9.)

However, in the twentieth century, vaccine development grew rapidly as scientific techniques advanced. Vaccines for deadly and widespread diseases such as diphtheria, pertussis, and tetanus were all developed before World War II (more on these diseases in Chapter 4).

Many more vaccines were developed in the second half of the twentieth century, including vaccines for polio, measles, mumps, and rubella (we'll talk about these in detail in Chapters 4 and 5). Some vaccines were very recently developed and added to the vaccination schedule, such as the human papillomavirus (HPV) vaccine for preteen girls and young women, approved in 2006 (see Chapter 6), and the most recent rotavirus vaccine for infants, approved in 2008 (see Chapter 4). Vaccine research is ongoing, and more new vaccines will be introduced in the future. Others may become obsolete. Many diseases that were once widespread are now rare in the United States, thanks to vaccination programs. Smallpox has been eradicated, and routine smallpox vaccines are no longer necessary. Polio and measles are the next diseases targeted for worldwide eradication. In the future, routine vaccinations for these diseases might not be necessary.

Vaccinating Facts

A small number of people in certain occupations still receive the smallpox vaccination. They include smallpox researchers working with the virus and health-care workers who might participate in mass vaccinations if smallpox were used as a biological weapon. Because the smallpox virus is no longer in the wild and the vaccine sometimes causes serious complications, it is no longer recommended for everyone.

The Least You Need to Know

◆ The first vaccine was created in the late 1700s to prevent smallpox.

◆ Routine smallpox vaccinations are no longer necessary because the disease has been eliminated worldwide.

◆ Some had social, religious, and personal objections to the first vaccine.

◆ It took almost 100 years for the second vaccine to be developed. Then, many more vaccines were created during the twentieth century.

Chapter 2

How Vaccines Work

In This Chapter

◆ Understanding biological threats to your body

◆ How your immune system works

◆ The role of vaccines in improving your immune system's response

◆ The characteristics of live and inactivated vaccines

◆ The benefits of herd immunity

Every day, you are under siege as numerous tiny biological invaders attack your body. Your body has developed a complex immune system to battle these substances and keep them from causing you harm. Without this immune system, you would not live long.

Vaccines work with your immune system to strengthen its protective response to two common types of harmful invaders: bacteria and viruses. The structures and functions of bacteria and viruses vary widely, so scientists have developed several different types of vaccines to help your immune system battle them and the diseases they can cause.

Bodily Threats

Bacteria and viruses are the two *pathogens* (disease-causing substances) that are most likely to make you sick. Fungi (such as molds) can also be pathogens that threaten your health. All of these pathogens can exist in soil, air, food, and water—all things you are exposed to and take in every day.

Luckily, your body can fight off many pathogens with its highly effective immune system, preventing or containing the many kinds of infections they can produce. Vaccines and medicines, such as *antibiotics*, can strengthen your body's immune response to certain pathogens, providing an extra layer of protection before or after an infection occurs.

Bacteria: Good and Bad

Several billion years old, bacteria are some of the oldest *organisms* known to science. A bacterium (the single form of the plural, "bacteria") is a single-celled organism—meaning it is made up of just one cell—with a very simple cell structure.

def•i•ni•tion

A **pathogen** is a biological substance capable of producing illness or disease in humans. The word "pathogen" originates from the Greek words *pathos*, meaning "suffering," and *gene*, meaning "to give birth to."

Antibiotics are substances that can inhibit the growth of or kill bacteria that cause certain infections. They do not work against illnesses that are caused by viruses.

An **organism** is a living thing that is one cell or larger and that can perform basic life functions, such as growing and reproducing. Every living thing, from a single-celled bacterium to a sunflower to an elephant, is an organism.

Many organisms' cells, such as human cells, have a more complex structure than that of single-celled bacteria. Complex cells are structured a bit like a chicken's egg. They include:

- A semipermeable membrane (similar to an egg shell) that lets the cell absorb and release materials

- A fluid called cytoplasm (similar to an egg white) that contains structures called organelles (which perform cell functions such as creating energy the cell needs)

- A nucleus (similar to an egg yolk) containing genetic information (the cell's blueprint) that tells the cell how to function

Bacteria, on the other hand, are so simple that their genetic information is not contained in a separate nucleus (they have no yolk). Also, some don't even have cell membranes (they have no shell).

Containing trillions of cells, your body is an extremely complex organism. Yet your body, and the natural world around you, relies on single-celled bacteria to properly function. You're never far from bacteria—in fact, they are on your skin and inside of you right now. For example, symbiotic (meaning helpful) bacteria live in your large intestine and help your body make vitamin K, a vitamin that helps your blood clot. In nature, bacteria help break down dead plant materials so they can be used again. Also, we use certain bacteria to turn milk into yogurt and cheese and to make antibiotics.

But, as you know by now, not all bacteria are helpful to humans. If the wrong bacteria get in the wrong part of your body, they can multiply rapidly and cause damage. The bacteria or their poisonous by-products, called toxins, can cause an infection. These bacteria usually damage your cells from the outside, but a few of the bacteria can enter your cells (getting through the shell) and damage them from within. Pathogenic bacteria can cause problems such as ear infections, strep throat, and tetanus.

 Health Advisory

Sometimes bacteria can cause outbreaks of food-borne illnesses that you might hear about on the news. Certain types of *salmonella* bacteria can infect meat or poultry and cause diarrhea and other problems. Certain types of *Escherichia coli* (*E. coli*) bacteria can contaminate food or water and sicken people.

Brain Booster _____

It is important to take antibiotics exactly as prescribed, even if you feel better before you finish taking all the medicine. If you don't, a few bacteria could survive and the illness could return or, worse, the bacteria could develop resistance to the medicine. Ultimately, the infection could become more difficult to treat.

Because bacterial cells are structured differently than your body's cells, antibiotics can often easily target and kill these cells. But some bacteria can very rapidly infect you and spread throughout your body, sometimes within just a few hours. By the time you take antibiotics to fight this type of bacteria, the infection might be too advanced for the drugs to work. A bacterium that can cause meningitis (*Neisseria meningitidis*) is an example of this type of bacteria.

Vaccinating Facts

Vaccines created to prevent dangerous bacterial infections include:

 ◆ The diphtheria, tetanus, and pertussis (whooping cough) vaccines
 ◆ The *Haemophilus influenzae* type b (Hib) vaccine
 ◆ The pneumococcal vaccine
 ◆ The meningococcal vaccine

Preventing dangerous bacterial infections with vaccinations is more effective than trying to treat them with antibiotics after you become infected.

Sneaky Viruses

Some viruses are harmless to humans, but others can make you very sick. Viruses have fewer parts than other pathogens; they are simply pieces of genetic material encased in a shell. Some experts believe that viruses are organisms; others do not, because viruses cannot function without help from another cell.

A virus functions by crossing your cells' membranes and taking over the cells from the inside, acting like tiny parasites (an organism that lives on or in another organism during part of its life cycle). From there, the virus forces the cells to make copies of the virus, and it usually kills or damages the healthy cell it takes over. The new copies of the virus then move on to take over other cells. This is why certain viruses can be so dangerous.

Different pathogenic viruses are spread in different ways. For example, a virus can be spread through the air via coughing and sneezing (such as the common cold virus), through insect bites (such as the West Nile virus), through contact with stool (such as the hepatitis A virus), or through sexual contact (such as the human immunodeficiency virus, or HIV). Some serious viruses can stay dormant (inactive) within a cell for many years before they *replicate*. Some viruses can damage a cell so much that the damaged cell begins to replicate abnormally; this can cause cancer.

def•i•ni•tion

Replication is a type of reproduction. When a virus or cell replicates, it creates more viruses or cells by making copies of itself.

Your immune system can usually handle and kill off mild viruses, such as a cold virus. But more serious viruses create a greater threat to your health. Antibiotics cannot stop viruses the way they can stop bacterial infections because antibiotics target parts of bacterial cells that viruses don't have.

Sometimes an antiviral medication can stop a virus from spreading by blocking some of the virus's processes, but these medications can damage healthy cells as well as infected ones. Also, like bacteria, viruses can mutate and become immune to medications. This is another reason why vaccines are so important. Ideally given before you can be infected with a virus, vaccines can strengthen your immune response to a virus so your body can more effectively fight it off.

Vaccinating Facts

Vaccines created to prevent dangerous viral infections include:

◆ The hepatitis B vaccine

◆ The rotavirus vaccine

◆ The polio vaccine

◆ The influenza vaccine

◆ The measles, mumps, and rubella (German measles) vaccines

◆ The varicella (chickenpox) vaccine

◆ The hepatitis A vaccine

◆ The human papillomavirus (HPV) vaccine

◆ The zoster (shingles) vaccine

Flexible Fungi

Like bacteria, fungi are naturally occurring organisms that can be either helpful or harmful to humans. Fungi can be single-celled, like bacteria, or they can be made up of many cells.

Common examples of fungi include mushrooms and yeasts, some of which we eat and use for cooking and alcohol fermentation. Other fungi, such as mold, help break down dead plant materials. Like bacteria, some fungi live on or in you, and helpful bacteria in your body keep these fungi from causing you any harm.

However, fungi can be problematic and cause infections in humans, such as athlete's foot or nail fungus (nail fungus is caused by a type of fungi called dermatophytes). Fungal infections are usually mild in people with normal immune systems. However, people with medical conditions such as AIDS or cancer, or who are taking certain medications such as steroids, can develop serious problems such as a fungal lung infection. Unfortunately, at this time, there are no vaccines to prevent fungal infections before they occur. The good news is there are medications available to help treat fungal infections and to ease symptoms associated with such infections.

Your Amazing Immune System

The first line of defense against pathogens is your body's complex immune system. To help understand how it works, think of your body as a walled city and your immune system as its defender and barrier from invaders.

Similar to a physical wall around a city, your skin and the mucous membranes that line the passageways into your body—such as your throat, lungs, and reproductive tract—are physical barriers against the pathogens trying to enter your body. Bacteria on your skin, for example, can't harm you unless you have an open cut or sore through which the bacteria can enter. Similarly, if someone with the cold virus coughs and you inhale some virus particles from the air, the mucous in your mouth, throat, and lungs are designed to make it difficult for the virus to enter further into your body and do any harm.

The Innate Immune System

So, what happens when a pathogen gets past your physical barriers? The white blood cells in what's called your innate immune system go to work and try to stop it. Red blood cells carry oxygen through your body, and your body's white blood cells fight off pathogens. A type of white blood cells called *phagocytes* constantly circulate in your blood and lymphatic (fluid drainage) system, patrolling for invaders like a guard patrolling the walls inside a city. Different types of white blood cells fight different types of pathogens.

When a pathogen enters your body and triggers a response from your immune system, the part of the pathogen that your immune system responds to is called an *antigen*. For example, suppose

def•i•ni•tion

Phagocytes are specialized white blood cells that find and consume pathogens and other foreign cells. They are part of the innate immune system.

An **antigen** is the part of a pathogen that causes an immune response. An antigen might be a part of the cell membrane on a bacterium, for example.

you scrape your knee and bacteria enter the cut. Your innate immune system then calls up a type of phagocytes, called neutrophils, that can fight bacteria by surrounding and dissolving the bacteria. As they do their job, neutrophils send out chemical signals to bring more immune system cells to the area to help them out. Blood and fluids build up in the area where the neutrophils are fighting. In response, the area where they are working can become red, swollen, and painful. So, when the cut on your knee swells up and hurts, this is a sign that your body is doing what it needs to do to fight infection.

Different types of white blood cells in the innate immune system are designed to attack different types of pathogens. The cells of the innate immune system patrol in the blood and stay near the physical barriers of the skin and mucous membranes so they can quickly respond to an invasion.

The Adaptive Immune System

The adaptive immune system is like a team of reinforcements that never forgets a battle. When your innate immune system cells can't destroy an antigen on their own, they send chemical signals to bring in the adaptive immune system's white blood cells, called lymphocytes. We'll discuss two types of lymphocytes: B cells and T cells.

B cells circulate in your bloodstream and have several branches dotted with substances called *antibodies*. These antibodies come in roughly 100 million different shapes to effectively "grab" different types of antigens when they encounter them. Most of these antibodies don't catch anything, because your body is not fighting off 100 million different types of invaders at once, but when they do catch an antigen, the B cell makes many copies of itself and its antibodies. These now-specialized B cells then release all their antibodies into your bloodstream to catch more of this antigen. In other words, B cells adapt to the threat they encounter by sending in reinforcements to fight it.

def•i•ni•tion

Part of the adaptive immune system, **antibodies** capture antigens and present them to T cells to be destroyed.

When an antibody in your bloodstream catches an antigen, immune system cells take it through the lymphatic system to a nearby lymph node, where there are lymphocytes called killer T cells. When an antibody is attached to an antigen, the killer T cell can then recognize and destroy the antigen. T cells cannot respond to an antigen unless an antibody is holding it, which demonstrates the importance of antibodies!

Vaccinating Facts

B cells get their name because they are created and mature in your bone marrow. T cells, while created by your bone marrow, mature in your thymus (an organ under your breast bone).

While the adaptive immune system is fighting off antigens, you might feel ill. Common symptoms of the viral disease influenza (the flu)—such as fever, body aches, and fatigue—are caused by your immune system's response to the virus. When you feel ill, your body is working to fight off an infection.

After the battle is won, most of the specialized B cells and T cells produced in the fight die off. Some of the specialized cells produced in battle, however, called memory cells, remain in the bloodstream, just in case that antigen returns. Because the cells are already customized to respond to the antigen, they are ready to go and can quickly stop the antigen from causing infections if it shows up again.

Vaccines at Work

Vaccines work by triggering a response from your adaptive immune system without actually causing a disease. A vaccine contains a disease-causing virus, bacterium, or bacterial toxin that has been killed or biologically changed, but that still causes your innate immune system to respond and call in your adaptive immune system for help. A vaccine does not make you sick with or give you the disease; it provides the immune system enough of the recognizable material from the pathogen to set in motion the protective response.

After your adaptive immune system destroys the modified antigen or antigens in a vaccine, the memory cells (some of those specialized B cells and T cells that were produced to fight the antigen) remain in your bloodstream. The presence of these memory cells is what gives you *immunity* against a pathogen.

def•i•ni•tion

You can develop **immunity** to certain diseases when your immune system has learned to recognize and destroy the pathogen that causes the disease. You can gain immunity to a disease in three ways: by catching and recovering from it, by inheriting or receiving protective antibodies (such as maternal antibodies that a mother passes on to her newborn child that provide short-term protection from a disease), or by getting vaccinated against the disease. Immunity to a disease can last for your whole lifetime or just for a few months to a few years, depending on the disease and the type of immunity you have.

Depending on the vaccine, these memory cells can remain in your body for a year, several years, or even your whole lifetime. As long as there are memory cells in your blood, you cannot become ill from that pathogen again—hence, you are immune to it.

Live Vaccines

The first vaccine for smallpox was a live vaccine, meaning it contained a live cowpox virus that triggered a relatively mild infection in humans. This infection, in turn, produced immunity to smallpox through the memory B cells and memory T cells the body had created.

Vaccinating Facts

Almost every live, attenuated vaccine used today prevents a viral infection. Inactivated (killed) vaccines work on a wider range of pathogens, preventing a number of viral and bacterial infections.

Today, to create a live vaccine, a virus is attenuated, meaning biologically weakened in a laboratory. Scientists can grow a virus in a laboratory in substances such as chicken cells. The virus is weakened to the point that it is unable to infect people, but it can still trigger an adaptive immune response. It is not capable of causing serious illness, and the antibodies to the virus will remain in the memory cells, creating immunity. Today, some vaccines are still created from a live virus or bacterium, including the measles, mumps, and rubella (MMR) vaccine; the varicella (chickenpox) vaccine; one type of influenza vaccine; and the zoster (shingles) vaccine (more on these in Chapters 5, 6, and 7).

Live vaccines are usually effective after just one dose, and immunity tends to last a long time. After vaccination with a live vaccine, however, you could pass on the weakened virus to someone else. Although this rarely occurs with the current live childhood vaccines, it did sometimes happen with the live version of the polio vaccine, which was later replaced by an inactivated version in the United States. If you receive a live vaccine and pass on the weakened virus to someone else, their healthy immune system could easily develop immunity to the weakened virus, just like you did. This process is called *contact immunity*.

def•i•ni•tion

> Contact immunity is a condition in which exposure to a weakened virus from household contact with a vaccinated person creates immunity. It is not a substitute for vaccination, but it can protect some unvaccinated people from disease. It has helped decrease outbreaks of polio during global vaccination campaigns.

But, if you or a household member has a very weakened immune system—for example, due to an immune system disorder or cancer treatments—the disease or a weakened version of it could develop after exposure to the vaccine (through vaccination or through household contact with a vaccinated person). Although this is quite rare, it can happen to some people.

So, you may be wondering, if live vaccines still have some health risks, why are they still used? The answer is that because live vaccines imitate a natural infection, they replicate and create a very robust immune response. Both memory B cells and memory T cells are involved in this response, which gives an infection very little chance of returning. Inactivated (killed) vaccines, on the other hand (which we'll explore in more detail in a minute), do not replicate inside your body. Therefore, the immune system's response to them is weaker, producing only memory B cells. Although inactivated vaccines are safe if you have a weakened immune system, they may be less effective or require more doses to create immunity than a live vaccine. Overall, a live vaccine is a more effective vaccine, which is why they are still used for certain diseases.

Inactivated Vaccines

Many modern vaccines use dead or disabled viruses or bacteria, as opposed to attenuated ones, to create immunity. These are called inactivated vaccines. The adaptive immune system still responds to these vaccines as if the pathogens are alive.

For example, the polio virus is killed chemically before it is used in its most common vaccine form, the inactivated polio vaccine (IPV). The immune system responds to the IPV and creates immunity. Because the IPV is killed and it does not replicate like the live oral polio vaccine (OPV) does, the immune response to the IPV is less robust than the immune response to the OPV. On the other hand, because the IPV virus is dead, there is no danger that this vaccine will cause polio even in people with weakened immune systems.

The diphtheria and tetanus vaccines are also inactivated vaccines. The bacteria that cause diphtheria and tetanus cause illness not by directly attacking cells, but rather by releasing a toxin that harms cells. To make vaccines for these illnesses, researchers first create and then inactivate the toxin, which is called a toxoid when it is inactivated. Toxoid vaccines can cause an immune response as if the bacteria are present, but cannot cause a disease. The vaccines for diphtheria, tetanus, and anthrax are all toxoid vaccines.

Some vaccines use just a piece of the bacteria or virus—such as its cell membrane or a piece of its genetic material—to trigger immunity. Examples of these vaccines are subunit vaccines and acellular vaccines, such as the acellular pertussis vaccine. Sometimes, the piece of the virus or bacteria must be linked to a biological carrier, such as a protein or a benign (or safe) version of a virus. This carrier then delivers the piece of the virus or bacteria to your immune system to trigger the response. Since these vaccines just contain a small piece of the pathogen, the pathogen cannot replicate like live vaccines can.

Because these inactivated vaccines cannot cause disease, they are generally safe, even if the recipient or a household member has an immune system problem. However, inactivated vaccines have some drawbacks. First of all, inactivated vaccines often require several doses to achieve full immunity. If you do not get all the recommended doses, you could still be vulnerable to the disease. Furthermore, some inactivated vaccines—such as the IPV—are slightly less effective, but are safer than live versions of the vaccine. Vaccine researchers and public health experts balance the risks and benefits of both live and inactivated vaccines when deciding which type works best and what is necessary to prevent each disease.

Achieving Herd Immunity

Although vaccinations have been proven to prevent many diseases, it is impossible to successfully vaccinate everyone. Both personal choice and individual circumstances prevent vaccination rates of 100 percent.

Some people simply cannot safely receive a vaccination that they might need. Certain medical conditions—for example, cancer or an immune system disorder—prevent some people from receiving certain vaccines. Pregnant women should not receive certain vaccines because the vaccines could harm the developing fetus. Others choose not to receive a vaccination because of social, medical, or religious concerns (more on this in Part 4). If vaccines are given in a series of doses, some people forget or are unable to get the entire series and do not achieve immunity to a disease. Also, vaccines themselves can fail to provide the necessary immunity. No vaccine comes with a 100 percent guaranteed success rate. Although 100 percent immunity to a disease is not possible, vaccines are certainly not all for naught. If enough people in a community are vaccinated against an infectious disease, *herd immunity* can protect the remaining

def•i•ni•tion

When a certain percentage of people in a community are vaccinated against a disease, they create **herd immunity** to the disease, which makes it unlikely that any unvaccinated members will catch the disease. Herd immunity is sometimes called "community immunity."

unvaccinated people. The vaccinations cause such a drop in the number of cases of a disease that it becomes less and less likely those unvaccinated will be exposed to the disease.

The percentage of vaccinated people required to create herd immunity in an area varies by disease. The very infectious disease measles requires about 95 percent of a population be vaccinated to achieve herd immunity. Vaccination rates for less infectious diseases can be lower to provide the benefit of herd immunity for unvaccinated people in a community.

If a large population achieves and maintains herd immunity against a disease, it is possible to completely eliminate the threat of the disease in that region. If this happens, sometimes the vaccination program for the disease can be discontinued in that area.

Health Advisory

Discontinuing a vaccination does not protect unvaccinated people from infectious diseases brought into the area by people from other regions. Also, if unvaccinated people travel to regions where a disease is prevalent, they could catch the disease.

Only one disease, smallpox, has been eliminated in the wild worldwide through a successful vaccination distribution program. For that reason, smallpox vaccination is no longer necessary for most people in the general population. Most likely, the next disease to be eliminated worldwide will be polio. At some point in the near future, polio vaccinations may become unnecessary as well.

The Least You Need to Know

◆ Vaccines help your body create immunity to harmful bacteria and viruses before you are exposed to them.

◆ Your innate and adaptive immune system work together to fend off harmful pathogens.

◆ B cells and T cells develop memory cells that remember and quickly stop pathogens they have fought before.

◆ Vaccines contain either live or inactivated pathogens, depending on the diseases they are designed to prevent.

◆ Herd immunity has the ability to protect unvaccinated people, and lead to the elimination of a disease threat and the need for its vaccine.

Chapter 3

Modern Vaccines

In This Chapter

- ◆ How clinical trials and other testing methods help make new vaccines safer
- ◆ Who makes recommendations about necessary vaccines
- ◆ Why the immunization schedule is so complex
- ◆ Why there are several different ways to administer a vaccine

The vaccines we know today are the product of many advances in science and technology. As a result, the number of vaccines on immunization schedules has increased dramatically over the past 20 years, with new technologies that have created new ways to deliver vaccines. Although most vaccines are still injected, there are newer, needle-free delivery methods—such as vaccine nasal sprays and jet injectors—now under development that can provide cheaper, safer, and more portable options for vaccinations.

From Smallpox to Today

A century ago, just five vaccines had been developed for smallpox, rabies, typhoid, cholera, and plague (the last three diseases are rarely seen today in the western world, thanks to improved sanitary conditions). By 1980, children were routinely vaccinated against seven diseases: diphtheria, pertussis (whooping cough), tetanus, polio, measles, mumps, and rubella. Today, children are routinely vaccinated against 14 different diseases before they even turn two. Needless to say, if you have children, you've probably noticed that they receive many more vaccinations than you did as a child.

In the twentieth century—especially the second half of the twentieth century—major scientific advances led to a better understanding of how bacteria, viruses, and the immune system work. Researchers used this knowledge to develop vaccines for a range of dangerous infectious diseases.

Vaccinating Facts

According to data from the CDC, before vaccines were created for these diseases, each year in the United States:

- Up to 20,000 people were paralyzed by polio.
- About 20,000 children developed serious problems such as meningitis or pneumonia from Hib infections.
- About 15,500 people died of diphtheria.
- About 9,000 people died from pertussis (whooping cough) infections.
- About 6,100 people died from invasive pneumococcal disease.
- Up to 2,100 infants died from congenital rubella syndrome.
- About 450 people died of measles.

Improved vaccine development methods made new and existing vaccines safer. In the late 1700s, Edward Jenner's original, cowpox-based smallpox vaccine carried the risk of passing on other diseases like tuberculosis from the human cowpox host. New scientific techniques, however, greatly decreased the risk of secondary infections from vaccinations.

Twentieth-century researchers learned how to purify live viruses, such as the vaccinia virus that creates immunity to smallpox, to make them safer. They learned how to create effective inactivated vaccines using just part of a bacterium or virus. Researchers added preservatives, stabilizers, and other substances to vaccines to prevent contamination by fungi and other pathogens, to extend the vaccines' shelf life, and to make the vaccines more effective. New techniques, such as freeze-drying, made vaccines more portable for wider distribution.

Modern vaccines are also a product of public and private collaboration. Federal public health agencies have funded vaccine research, coordinated human testing of new vaccines, and regulated the quality and safety of vaccines. Private groups, such as the March of Dimes, raised funds for vaccine development and promoted vaccine distribution. Private manufacturers make the vaccines you might get today.

How Vaccines Are Developed

Even if there is a great need for a vaccine and a researcher has an idea about how to create one, it can take 10 years or longer for a vaccine to go from concept to your doctor's office. Potential vaccines go through a long process of development, testing, and licensing before they ever reach you. Both old and new vaccines are continuously monitored after they are licensed to make sure they are safe and effective.

To create a vaccine for a disease, researchers first need to study and understand how that disease causes illness. Why does one virus cause disease in humans when another virus does not? Does the disease-causing bacterium or its toxic by-products sicken people? How does the human immune system respond to a pathogen? Researchers conduct basic scientific research to understand how and why a pathogen causes disease. Once they understand this, they can work on a potential vaccine.

The next step is testing this knowledge with laboratory tests and computer models. Computer models can simulate how the immune system works, and look at how human antibodies might respond to certain antigens. Researchers use this data to create a vaccine that they hope will safely prevent the disease.

Next, the vaccine is ready for testing on animals. These tests focus on the safety of the vaccine, and researchers look for any problems that the vaccines cause in animals. If animals respond well to the vaccine, it is tested on humans in three-stage clinical trials.

Clinical Trials

There are three phases of human clinical trials for vaccines. Phase I clinical trials involve a small group of people (generally fewer than 100 people) who meet certain criteria and who volunteer to receive the experimental vaccine. They are monitored to see whether the vaccine causes any health problems at certain dosages. Because these trials are very small, involving few people, they only provide data on any extremely common side effects or health problems caused by the vaccine, such as muscle aches. Phase I clinical trials are designed to test the general safety of a vaccine, and to see how effective it might be.

Brain Booster

In 1974, the U.S. Congress passed the National Research Act to make sure that people who participate in medical research are treated ethically. The new law created a commission of experts who set policies on how to conduct medical research. These experts make sure that people have access to clinical trials, that they understand the risks and benefits of the trial, and that their health is protected.

When Phase I results are positive, a Phase II clinical trial is designed for implementation. These trials test how well the vaccine creates immunity in several hundred people, and what dosage is most effective, while continuing to monitor volunteers for safety.

If the results are good in Phase II, a Phase III study is designed for the vaccine to learn how well it works on greater numbers of people and to further check for any safety problems. Phase III studies are very large, often involving thousands or tens of thousands of people and done over months or years. The studies take place among volunteers at many different medical centers, sometimes located in different countries.

For example, a Phase III study of the rotavirus vaccine (currently used to prevent a sometimes-fatal gastrointestinal disease in infants) included over 68,000 infants. Half the infants were given a *placebo*, and the other half received the actual vaccine being studied. Researchers then compared the number of side effects in those who received a placebo to those who received the vaccine.

def•i•ni•tion

A **placebo** is a harmless substance that is given to someone in place of a vaccine or medication in clinical trials. Researchers sometimes compare the health outcomes of the people who received a placebo to those who received the vaccine or medication being investigated.

Phase III trials of vaccines ask the question, "How well does this vaccine provide protection against a disease in a wide variety of people?" To answer this question, researchers need the best possible and most conclusive data about the vaccine. Ideally, Phase III trials have two important components that prevent any human bias that could make the data less accurate:

◆ They are randomized control trials (RCTs). An RCT randomly assigns who will receive the new vaccine, called the experimental group, and who will not, called the control group. Usually a computer generates this information. The control group might receive a placebo, or (if a new version of an existing vaccine is being tested) the control group might receive the current version of the vaccine. The new vaccine or the control substance is distributed evenly across all groups of participants, regardless of their gender, health, or other categories. This strategy provides good data on how many different kinds of people would respond to the new vaccine.

◆ They are double-blind, which means that neither the patients nor the people who give them the substance know whether or not a patient received the new vaccine or a placebo (this information is revealed at the end of the study). The patients can't pressure the researcher to receive the new vaccine, and the patients and researchers are less likely to be biased in how they report and analyze the data. For example, a patient (or his parent) who knows he received the new vaccine might report a fever. But if he knows he received the placebo, he might not report the fever.

Phase III trials are the last big test before a vaccine might be licensed for distribution to the public. It is important to construct the trial so that it provides the best data possible. Phase III trials should include as many volunteers as possible, to get the best information on rare side effects or other problems from the vaccine.

Clinical Trial Phases

Phase	No. of People in Trial	Goal of Trial
I	Less than 100	Check for safety/side effects
II	Up to 300	Check for immunity from vaccine and best dosage
III	1,000 or more	Test how well vaccine prevents disease in a large number of people

Licensing and Monitoring Vaccines

If the vaccine appears safe and effective after all of the clinical trials are done, the manufacturer applies for a license from the U.S. Food and Drug Administration (FDA). The FDA reviews the clinical trial data and examines the manufacturing facility where the vaccine will be made. If the data and the facility pass the inspection, the vaccine is licensed for use.

Clinical trials provide good information about whether a vaccine is safe and effective. If a vaccine creates very rare side effects or has other rare problems, however, these issues might not show up in a clinical trial. For example, if a vaccine is tested on 10,000 people in clinical trials but it causes a rare side effect in every 500,000 people, this side effect probably would not show up in clinical trials. For example, an earlier version of the rotavirus vaccine sometimes caused a rare but serious intestinal problem called intussusception. This problem did not appear in Phase III trials because the trial was not large enough to show this data (the old rotavirus vaccine was withdrawn from the market in 1999 and is no longer used today). New rotavirus vaccines were tested in much larger trials to check for these rare side effects.

For this reason, after a vaccine is licensed, it is monitored for any problems. If a patient becomes ill after receiving a vaccine, the illness is reported to the Vaccine Adverse Events Reporting System (VAERS), a monitoring system explained in more detail in Chapter 14. Every time the manufacturer makes a batch of vaccines, called a "lot," the vaccines are tested for safety, purity, and effectiveness. If there is a problem with the lot, the FDA can recall that lot of the vaccine.

> **Vaccinating Facts**
>
> The monitoring period of licensed vaccines is sometimes called Phase IV of the clinical trial. Although the vaccine is available for use at that point, it could be recalled if there is a pattern of safety problems.

The Immunization Schedule

The Centers for Disease Control and Prevention (CDC) publishes a Recommended Immunization Schedule listing recommended vaccines for newborns through children 6 years old, children 7 through 18 years old, and adults. The schedule explains the following:

- ◆ What vaccinations are recommended for every age group

- ◆ How many doses of the vaccine are required to ensure immunity to the disease

- ◆ How to space out the doses

- ◆ Who should or should not receive the vaccine (for example, some vaccines are not safe for pregnant women)

The recommended vaccination schedule needs some flexibility to accommodate certain patient needs. For that reason, the CDC also publishes other vaccine information, such as a schedule for catch-up immunizations (for children who missed some childhood vaccinations) and an immunization schedule for adults with certain health conditions (who might need to postpone or even forgo some vaccinations).

These immunization schedules are updated annually, with each year's new schedule published in January. Yearly updates are important for a variety of reasons. A new vaccine, such as the recently licensed human papillomavirus (HPV) vaccine, might be approved and added to the schedule. A new combination vaccine might become available, which combines several different vaccines into one shot and can replace some individual vaccines. Or, recommendations for the use of a vaccine might change. For example, the yearly influenza vaccine used to be recommended for children ages 6 months to 5 years old; in 2009, the recommendation changed to include children ages 6 months to 18 years old.

Brain Booster

The current recommended vaccination schedules for children, adolescents, and adults are available at the CDC online at www.cdc.gov/vaccines/recs/schedules/default.htm.

Who Recommends Vaccines?

The federally appointed Advisory Committee on Immunization Practices (ACIP) makes recommendations to the CDC on adding vaccines to the immunization schedules each year or changing existing vaccine recommendations. ACIP is made up of a group of 15 vaccination experts, as well as a number of nonvoting members, chosen by the U.S. Department of Health and Human Services. Each ACIP member serves for up to four years on the committee. After a vaccine is licensed, ACIP provides advice on how to use the vaccine and related substances (such as immune globulin, a blood product). The group meets three times a year, and most ACIP meetings are open to the public.

The Committee on Infectious Diseases (COID) is made up of members of the American Academy of Pediatrics (AAP). These doctors follow any new developments in infectious diseases, and make recommendations about vaccine policy to other members of the AAP. The AAP is involved in vaccine recommendations because so many vaccines are recommended for children.

The American Academy of Family Physicians (AAFP), a group of doctors who treat both children and adults, also has a committee that evaluates vaccines, called the Commission on Clinical Policies and Research (CCPR). The CCPR provides recommendations to its members on adding vaccines to the schedules or changing current vaccination recommendations.

Recommendations made by the COID and the CCPR usually follow the ACIP's recommendations. Sometimes, however, the COID and the CCPR make slightly different recommendations for their doctors to follow.

Vaccinating Facts

Once a vaccine is added to the vaccination schedule, individual states decide whether to require the vaccine in order for children or young adults to attend school. If your child cannot receive a vaccination for medical reasons, however, you can opt out of it and he or she can still attend school. Learn more about vaccination requirements and exemptions in Chapter 13.

Not surprisingly, the current vaccination schedule is very complex. If a vaccine is added to the schedule, ACIP must decide how to add the vaccine to the schedule so that the doses of the vaccine do not interfere with the effectiveness of other vaccines on the schedule. The committee also needs to decide how the vaccine might fit into the schedule for the recommended well-child visits. Lastly, they need to decide how or if these recommendations apply to people with certain health problems.

Other issues also affect decisions about the vaccine schedule, such as whether the vaccine is cost-effective (saves money in future health-care costs) and whether someone can safely receive doses of two different brands of one vaccine. All of these factors combined make vaccine recommendations a complicated process.

Alternative Vaccination Schedules

Some vaccines on the childhood vaccination schedule are combined together into one injection, such as the four-dose diphtheria, tetanus, and acellular pertussis (DTaP) vaccine and the two-dose measles, mumps, and rubella (MMR) vaccine. If vaccines such as MMR were given separately, your child would need many more shots to achieve immunity to the diseases. For example, if the MMR vaccine was split into individual vaccines, your child would need six shots rather than two shots to gain immunity to these diseases. Combination vaccines are increasingly popular because they are convenient and reduce the number of shots needed. Newer combination vaccines include a DTaP and *Haemophilus influenzae* type b (Hib) combination vaccine and a DTaP, hepatitis B, and polio combination vaccine.

You may have heard about alternative vaccination schedules for children that split up combination vaccines into individual vaccines. Some people are interested in alternative vaccination schedules because they believe they are safer for their children. They might want to delay or split up vaccinations so that their child will receive fewer antigens at once, to alleviate concerns that are addressed in Part 4 of this book. Alternative schedules involve many more shots for children and often would involve many more doctor's office visits to get the shots.

Health Advisory

Merck & Company, the only U.S. manufacturer of the MMR vaccine, recently announced that they might stop making individual measles, mumps, and rubella vaccines. Parents and providers who want to follow an alternative vaccination schedule might not have access to individual vaccines. This could put their children at even greater risk for vaccine-preventable diseases, if the parents do not want their children to receive the MMR vaccine.

The committees that make recommendations about the vaccination schedule base their advice on the latest scientific research and knowledge. Each childhood vaccine is given at a specific time to create immunity to a disease before a child might be exposed to it. Alternative vaccination schedules can result in delays in vaccination, making children vulnerable to sometimes-fatal, vaccine-preventable diseases.

Any change to the recommended childhood vaccination schedule, either by choice or circumstance (such as a serious illness that requires postponing the vaccination for a few months), increases that child's dependence on the herd immunity of the people around him or her. If his or her classmates, family members, and other community members are adequately immunized against a disease, he or she should be protected from the disease as well. If others are not vaccinated, however, he or she is vulnerable to catching the disease. Alternative vaccination schedules only provide protection if everyone else follows the standard vaccination schedule.

Vaccine Delivery

Vaccination delivery strategies can change over time as advances are made in science, as more people are vaccinated, and as the risks of catching a disease change.

For instance, the first polio vaccine, licensed for use in the United States in 1955, was an inactivated vaccine (IPV) created by researcher Jonas Salk. Although the vaccine was effective and could not cause polio, researcher Albert Sabin believed that a live, attenuated vaccine would work better. Sabin developed and promoted the live oral (taken by mouth) polio vaccine (OPV), which replaced the IPV in the 1960s.

The OPV was more effective at preventing polio, a common and greatly feared disease, than the IPV. But like other live vaccines, it carried a very slight risk of causing disease in the recipient. According to the CDC, the OPV caused polio in about 1 of every 2.4 million people who were vaccinated with it. Nonetheless, the OPV was used in the United States from the 1960s to the late 1990s. If you were a child then, you probably received the OPV to prevent polio.

As polio rates decreased, thanks to nationwide vaccination programs, and the IPV's effectiveness increased with improved vaccine creation techniques, the U.S. government decided to recommend the lower-risk IPV over the higher-risk OPV. This is why children in the United States today receive the inactivated (injected) IPV rather than the live (oral) OPV.

Injected and Oral Vaccines

Vaccine delivery methods can also vary depending on the resources available in each country. Increasingly, delivery methods that work in wealthier countries need to be changed to achieve high vaccination rates in developing countries.

Today, most vaccines in the United States are given by injection. It is a convenient and quick way to provide vaccinations. Injected vaccines do have some disadvantages. The injection itself can be painful, and you might feel sore at the injection site for a while. Some people don't like needles and will skip a vaccination to avoid an injection.

An injected vaccine needs to be given by a health-care professional, and it requires a supply of sterile needles. Injected and oral vaccines must be refrigerated until they are used, and injected vaccines can be expensive to manufacture. These requirements are not a problem in the United States, but medical care, medical equipment, and reliable electricity for refrigeration are sometimes hard to find in the developing world.

> ### Vaccinating Facts
>
> Most vaccines must be kept within a certain cold temperature range in their journey from the manufacturer to the patient. The system of transporting and storing vaccines at the right temperature is called a cold chain. If the cold chain is broken and a vaccine becomes too warm or too cold while it travels or while it is stored, then it becomes ineffective and won't create immunity.

A few vaccines are given orally in the United States and elsewhere. The rotavirus vaccine—a live vaccine given to infants to prevent infection by a virus that causes diarrhea and dehydration—is an oral vaccine. Oral vaccines are designed to survive the trip through your stomach without being destroyed by stomach acid. They create immunity in the mucous membranes of your small intestine, part of your immune system's physical defenses. This causes a stronger immune response than injected vaccines, which bypass your first line of defense. Because oral vaccines don't require special equipment (such as sterile needles) to administer them, oral vaccines can be useful in areas of the world with limited access to health care.

Other Delivery Methods

Because needle-free vaccine delivery systems offer many advantages, researchers are testing a number of new techniques. The live, attenuated influenza vaccine (LAIV), for example, which is designed to prevent the yearly flu in people aged 2 through 49, is given by nasal spray (an injected, inactivated version is also available). Specially designed jet injectors are being developed that could provide quick vaccinations without needles. These hand-held devices work by using air pressure to push the vaccine past the skin's barrier. If there were a large outbreak of a disease, a jet injector could provide quick and sterile injections for many people. Also, skin patches called transcutaneous vaccines are being researched to deliver some vaccines.

Edible vaccines, which are still in the trial stage, could particularly benefit the developing world. With edible vaccines, food such as a potato, tomato, or banana is genetically engineered to grow certain disease antigens that can cause an immune response. When the food is eaten, the immune system responds to the antigens, creating immunity to a disease. These genetically engineered foods could be grown inexpensively in the countries that need certain vaccines. Researchers are also investigating the use of edible bacteria, used to make yogurt and cheese, to deliver vaccines to the body.

How Long Does Immunity Last?

It's not always easy to tell how long a vaccination will provide protection against a disease. If the disease is relatively rare, such as polio, a vaccinated person is fairly unlikely to encounter it and "test" his or her immunity. Unless there is an outbreak of a disease among a population of vaccinated and unvaccinated people, it can be hard to measure how long a vaccination might last. Researchers might not yet know how long newer vaccines will provide immunity because there is not yet enough data available.

Furthermore, not every vaccine needs to provide lifelong protection. Some childhood vaccines, such as the rotavirus vaccine, only need to provide protection for a few years while a young child is in the greatest danger of becoming seriously ill from the disease.

In general, however, live attenuated vaccines provide protection against a disease for a longer time than inactivated vaccines. Some live vaccines, such as the measles vaccine, are believed to provide lifelong protection from disease. Inactivated vaccines, on the other hand, sometimes require periodic booster shots to remain effective. The influenza vaccine, live or inactivated, provides protection for just one year because the viruses that cause influenza mutate frequently.

The Least You Need to Know

- All new vaccines go through an extensive testing and approval process prior to public distribution.
- Medical experts create and update the CDC's vaccination schedules.
- Alternative vaccination schedules can expose your child to disease.
- Most vaccines are injected, but several needle-free vaccination methods are now in use or are being developed.

Part 2

Standard Vaccinations for Every Age

This part covers the many childhood and adolescent vaccinations recommended today, and why it is important to get these vaccinations at certain ages. It also describes the vaccines and boosters recommended for adults and seniors. Lastly, it explains what vaccines you might need if you have an acute or chronic illness.

Chapter 4

Vaccinations in the First Year of Life

In This Chapter

- The seven vaccine series recommended from birth to one year

- The importance of getting vaccines early in life

- How a child might respond to different vaccines

- Criteria for not receiving certain vaccines

Babies literally start receiving vaccinations from the day they are born. One vaccine is administered just after birth. Over the course of their first year, babies receive vaccinations against a total of nine different diseases. It may seem like a lot for such tiny bodies to handle, but these vaccinations are necessary so early in life because the viral and bacterial diseases they prevent are often much more harmful and permanently debilitating to infants and young children than to adults. Furthermore, if a baby or young child does catch a vaccine-preventable disease, the treatment options are often limited at such a young age.

> **Health Advisory** _____
>
> If your child has a life-threatening reaction to a dose of any vaccine, he or she will not receive anymore doses of it. If he or she has a life-threatening reaction to a vaccine ingredient, such as a preservative, he or she might need to avoid other vaccinations as well. Signs of a life-threatening reaction can include breathing problems, choking, and/or the sudden onset of an itchy face, hives, swelling, or stomach pain.
>
> Before your child receives any vaccination, tell your doctor if your child has had any severe reactions to previous vaccinations or is somewhat or very ill with an acute illness. The vaccination might need to be postponed until your child is feeling better.

Many childhood vaccines have been improved over the years, decreasing the chance of side effects in young children. The vaccines your child receives today are the products of many years of scientific research and study. Now that you understand how vaccines work, as explained in Chapter 2, let's explore what vaccines babies receive in their first year of life.

Hepatitis B

The first vaccine a baby ever receives, often within a few hours of being born, is the hepatitis B vaccine. The vaccine protects them from the very contagious and dangerous hepatitis B virus that attacks the liver, a critical bodily organ.

The liver creates substances that help you digest food and help your blood clot. It also filters toxic chemicals from your blood, stores important vitamins and minerals such as iron, and stores sugars that your body uses for energy, among other roles. Your liver can be injured by viruses, bacteria, and toxic chemicals such as alcohol. They can all cause liver inflammation, which is called hepatitis. When a liver becomes inflamed, it can't perform all of its critical roles for the circulatory and digestive systems. As a result, someone with hepatitis can develop symptoms such as jaundice (yellowing of skin and eyes), nausea, fatigue, loss of appetite, and stomach problems. Sometimes, hepatitis can lead to chronic liver problems or liver cancer.

Because viruses are the most common cause of hepatitis, two vaccines have been developed to prevent two types of viral hepatitis. One is the hepatitis A vaccine, which we'll discuss more in Chapter 5 because it is usually given to children in their second year of life; the second is the hepatitis B vaccine, typically given at birth.

Hepatitis B can be either an acute or a chronic infection. Acute hepatitis has the ability to go away by itself without harm, but chronic hepatitis B can permanently damage the liver. An acute hepatitis B infection can sometimes turn into a chronic infection. So, either way, hepatitis B can be very dangerous—especially to infants. (See Chapter 8 for more on acute and chronic illnesses.)

Brain Booster _____

Children who catch hepatitis B when they are under age five are far more likely to develop a chronic hepatitis B infection than adults who catch the virus.

Hepatitis B is spread by contact with an infected person's bodily fluids, such as blood. People at risk for catching hepatitis B include intravenous drug users, hemodialysis (a method for removing certain substances from blood) patients, health-care workers, and people who have had sexual relations with someone who is infected with the hepatitis B virus. Hepatitis B can be medically managed, but it cannot be cured once you have it.

Brain Booster _____

Hepatitis C, D, and E viruses exist as well. All are usually spread by contact with the bodily fluids or stool of an infected person and tend to cause similar symptoms, including nausea, fatigue, and jaundice. Unfortunately, no vaccine is available to prevent hepatitis C, which can become chronic and damage the liver. Hepatitis D and E are rare in the United States.

Despite these known risk factors for hepatitis B infection, many people who have hepatitis B do not fit in any of the risk categories. This may be because hepatitis B is very contagious, and because it can live outside the body for a week. Furthermore, an infected person might feel healthy for months or even years before he or she has any symptoms of the disease. Also, people often don't know they have hepatitis B and unknowingly pass it on to others.

The hepatitis B vaccine is an inactivated vaccine. It was licensed in the United States in 1986, and it is available for children as a single vaccine (which must be used for the first dose) or as a combination vaccine (which can be used for later doses). One combination vaccine includes the hepatitis B and *Haemophilus influenzae* type b (Hib) vaccines. Another combination includes the hepatitis B vaccine; the diphtheria, tetanus, and acellular pertussis (DTaP) vaccine; and the polio vaccine (more on all of these other vaccines later in this chapter).

Why Now?

Most infants receive a hepatitis B vaccination within a day of their birth, and this is the only vaccine that is given to infants just after birth. They are vaccinated so quickly because if a pregnant woman has hepatitis B, it is quite likely she will pass it on to her infant during birth. This is true for both vaginal and cesarean births. Because the hepatitis B virus *incubates* in the body for a month or longer before it develops into disease, rapid vaccination can prevent the infection from developing in a baby. Infants who catch hepatitis B from their mothers have a 90 percent chance of developing the chronic, more damaging version of the virus.

def•i•ni•tion

You don't get sick the moment pathogenic viruses or bacteria enter your bloodstream. It takes a while for the pathogen to **incubate,** which means it reproduces and spreads throughout your body. After this incubation period, you start to have symptoms. A vaccination given during the incubation period of a virus can sometimes stop or slow down the growth of the pathogens.

What to Expect

To create immunity to hepatitis B, infants are usually given three shots over a six-month period as follows:

- The first shot is usually given within 12 hours of birth.

- The second shot is given at one or two months of age, and sometimes another shot is given at the four-month doctor's visit if it is part of a combination vaccine.

- The third shot is given at 6 months of age, but it can be given as late as 18 months.

If the mother has hepatitis B, the newborn infant also receives a shot of hepatitis B *immune globulin* within 12 hours of birth.

def•i•ni•tion

If a child or adult needs temporary immunity to a disease to protect them until they are fully vaccinated, they might get a shot of **immune globulin**. This is a blood product that contains antibodies that may help protect you against the disease for a few months.

After getting the shots, crying is a given, but an infant also might have soreness at the injection site or develop a fever. While getting shots is never fun for infants (or anyone!), the hepatitis B vaccine is believed to provide lifelong protection against the virus.

Who Might Not Get It

A child should not receive the vaccine if he or she has a severe allergy to baker's yeast because yeast cells are used to make the hepatitis B vaccine. A child's health-care provider should be advised if there is a history of allergies to baker's yeast in the family so the risks and benefits of the vaccine in light of the family's medical history can be discussed. If an infant has a severe reaction to the birth dose of hepatitis B, he or she should not receive anymore doses of the vaccine.

Rotavirus

Rotaviruses are a group of common viruses that can cause fever, vomiting, stomach cramps, and diarrhea. Rotavirus is usually spread by contact with an infected person's stool. By age two, almost all children have been infected with a rotavirus.

In most cases, the illness lasts up to eight days and then goes away on its own. Sometimes, however, severe diarrhea from a rotavirus infection can cause dehydration, or a decreased amount of fluids in the body. Signs of dehydration in an infant include sunken eyes, lethargy, irritability, dry skin, and a dry diaper. Untreated dehydration can be very dangerous, and a dehydrated infant needs immediate medical attention. Sometimes, an infant will need to be hospitalized to receive intravenous fluids (delivered directly into the blood by a needle inserted into a vein).

A vaccine designed to provide protection against many rotaviruses was approved in 1998, but it was removed from the market in 1999 and it is no longer available. This vaccine was linked to a rare bowel problem called intussusception, in which part of the bowel folds back upon itself and causes a painful obstruction. When intussusception occurs, it needs prompt medical attention because it can be fatal if untreated. It occurs naturally in about 1 out of every 2,000 to 3,000 infants, but it occurred more often in infants who received the 1998 vaccine.

Two different rotavirus vaccines were licensed in 2006 and 2008, and studies have found no link between these vaccines and intussusception. Today, your infant will receive one of these two new vaccines. They are both live attenuated vaccines, given by mouth to infants. The 2006 vaccine requires three doses to create immunity, and the 2008 vaccine requires two doses.

Health Advisory

Rotavirus and many other infectious diseases are often spread by your hands. Always wash your hands after using the bathroom, helping a child use the bathroom, changing a diaper, before making or eating food, before and after you bandage a cut, and before and after you help someone who is sick. Wash your hands after you cough, sneeze, or blow your nose, and after you handle garbage, animals, or animal waste. Use warm running water and soap for at least 20 seconds. Alcohol-based hand sanitizers are also effective when soap and water aren't available.

The two new rotavirus vaccines are about 75 percent effective at preventing any rotavirus infections. They are over 95 percent effective at preventing severe rotavirus infections that require hospitalization.

Because these two vaccines are quite new, their long-term effects are still being studied. There is less data available about them than about vaccines that have been around for a long time, such as the measles and polio vaccines. Because of the link between intussusception and previous versions of the rotavirus vaccine, however, newer rotavirus vaccines went through extensive clinical trials before they were approved. They are currently being closely monitored for both safety and effectiveness.

Why Now?

When babies are born, their blood contains their mother's antibodies, which protect them from diseases to which their mothers are immune. These maternal antibodies only provide temporary protection, however, which gradually fades during children's first year of life. Several multi-dose childhood vaccinations, including the rotavirus vaccination, are begun when babies are two months old. By the time the babies are six months old, they have enough doses of these vaccines to be immune to the disease, and they no longer need maternal antibodies.

The rotavirus vaccine is the only live vaccine babies receive until they reach 12 months or older and all the maternal antibodies have left their blood. When maternal antibodies are present in a baby's blood, they could make a live vaccine less effective. Maternal rotavirus antibodies can decline quickly, however, because natural rotavirus infection is still common in unvaccinated children as young as four months old. So, giving the live vaccine early on helps pick up where the maternal antibodies appear to leave off. In addition, the live rotavirus vaccine is given orally (rather than injected), so it creates immunity in the gut.

The rotavirus vaccination series usually starts when an infant is two months old, and it is generally finished by the time the baby is six months old. It is important to create immunity quickly because infants are most likely to develop rotavirus infections between ages three months and three years. Also, children in child care centers are at a higher risk of exposure to rotavirus than those at home.

The rotavirus vaccine is typically recommended for preterm infants as well, once they reach at least six weeks old.

What to Expect

In general, infants should receive the rotavirus vaccine at two, four, and six months of age for one vaccine brand, or at two and four months of age for the other vaccine brand. The first dose can be given as early as six weeks after birth, however, and doses can be as close as four weeks apart instead of two months apart. An infant should receive all of the doses by the time he or she is eight months old. Both rotavirus vaccines were licensed with this age restriction to decrease the chance of intussusception, which is more common in older children. To reach this target, the vaccination series must begin by the time the infant is 15 weeks old. If an infant spits out the dose, the doctor will not repeat the dose that day. Instead, the infant will receive the next dose as scheduled.

While the rotavirus vaccines do not have any known serious side effects, they can cause some mild symptoms such as diarrhea or vomiting and can also make an infant irritable. Like the yearly influenza virus, rotavirus rates increase in the wintertime. The doctor might decide to follow an accelerated schedule (like one dose a month) if the winter season is approaching.

Who Might Not Get It

Children with a latex allergy should not receive the two-dose rotavirus vaccine since the applicator of this brand of the vaccine contains latex. Those who have had intussusception might need to avoid the rotavirus vaccination altogether. Also, the vaccination might be postponed if a child has recently received a blood product or a blood transfusion.

It's important to discuss vaccinations options with a doctor if a child has a weakened immune system caused by a disease (such as cancer) or drug treatment (such as steroids), or if he or she has chronic digestive problems.

Diphtheria, Tetanus, and Acellular Pertussis (DTaP)

Diphtheria, tetanus, and pertussis (also known as whooping cough) are all bacterial diseases. Most of these diseases' symptoms are caused by toxins released by the bacteria, not by the bacteria themselves. The vaccines for diphtheria and tetanus are toxoid vaccines; they are created by inactivating the toxins and using them to trigger an immune response. Pertussis is an acellular vaccine (it does not contain whole cells of the bacterium).

Diphtheria is contagious, and is usually spread through coughing and sneezing. It can cause breathing and swallowing problems due to a build-up of mucus in the throat, and can also damage the heart or nervous system, among other things. Diphtheria is fatal for about 20 percent of children under five years of age who catch it. But, thanks to vaccinations, diphtheria is now extremely rare in the United States.

Vaccinating Facts

The Iditarod is a yearly dogsled race along the Iditarod Trail that runs from Anchorage, Alaska, to Nome, Alaska. In 1925, when there was a diphtheria outbreak in Nome, the Iditarod Trail was used to deliver lifesaving diphtheria serum (a blood product that was used to prevent diphtheria before a vaccine was developed) from Anchorage to Nome. A series of relay teams of dogs and their drivers (called *mushers*) carried the serum over 700 miles in less than a week, braving a blizzard during the last two legs. There is a statue of Balto, the lead dog during the blizzard, in New York City's Central Park.

Tetanus comes from spores of the tetanus bacterium often found in soil and animal feces. If they enter the blood, usually through a puncture wound or scratch, they can grow into bacteria whose toxins can cause severe muscle spasms. These muscle spasms (sometimes called *lockjaw*) can affect the throat and cause sometimes-fatal breathing problems. Newborn babies can get neonatal tetanus if they don't have maternal antibodies to it (that is, if their mother is not vaccinated against tetanus) and their umbilical cord becomes infected. Yet (unlike diphtheria) tetanus is not contagious, so someone with tetanus cannot give it to another person.

Brain Booster

Contrary to popular belief, rust does not cause tetanus. If you step on a rusty nail, however, and it punctures your skin, you could develop tetanus if you are not adequately vaccinated against it. This is because dirt that contains tetanus bacterium spores could be on the rusty nail.

Pertussis is contagious, and is often spread from adults to young children through coughing and sneezing. It is more dangerous in children and infants than in adults, and young children who catch it can suffer from frightening, sometimes deadly coughing and choking spells. Pertussis can also cause seizures and pneumonia.

The diphtheria, tetanus, and pertussis vaccines are usually combined into one shot, called the diphtheria, tetanus, and acellular pertussis (DTaP) vaccination. Because it takes five doses of each vaccine over several years to achieve immunity, if given separately, a child would need to get 15 different shots. Immunizing through the combination vaccine only requires five total shots.

The current DTaP vaccination series was licensed for use in the United States in 1997. An older version of the combination vaccine—called the diphtheria, tetanus, and pertussis (DTP) vaccine—had a fairly high rate of side effects from the pertussis component, which used whole cells of the toxin to create immunity. Some children who received the vaccine cried inconsolably for several hours after the vaccination, developed a high fever, or had seizures. To help prevent these problems, the pertussis component of the vaccine was reformulated to use just a piece of the pertussis bacteria—called an acellular pertussis vaccine—rather than a whole cell. This change to the vaccine greatly decreased the chances of these side effects. Children who still cannot tolerate the pertussis part of the vaccine can receive the diphtheria and tetanus (DT) vaccine that contains just the diphtheria and tetanus toxoids.

> **Vaccinating Facts**
>
> While vaccines have scientific and sometimes complicated names, thankfully most of them are referred to by an acronym—such as DTaP or MMR—to make them easier to reference and remember.

Why Now?

Diphtheria and pertussis are highly contagious and are especially harmful to infants and young children (more so than adults). Also, tetanus spores are in the environment all around us, making it virtually impossible to control exposure to them. It's important to start the vaccination series for DTaP at a young age to ensure protection against these once-feared diseases as soon as possible.

The protective effect of maternal antibodies that an infant receives from his or her mother fade over the course of the child's first year of life. An infant needs several doses of the DTaP vaccine by six months to begin to create his or her own lasting immunity to these diseases.

What to Expect

The DTaP vaccination is a series of shots given in five doses between two months and six years of age. A child will receive a dose at 2 months, 4 months, 6 months, 15 to 18 months (in some cases, the fourth dose is given at 12 months), and finally between ages 4 and 6.

After each shot, a child might have a fever or redness, swelling, or soreness at the injection site. These side effects are more common after the fourth or fifth shot. Within a few days of the shot, a child might be fussy or tired, eat less, or vomit. About 1 in 1,000 children cries inconsolably for several hours afterward. Seizures and high fever are possible, but are much less common (about 1 in 14,000 and 16,000, respectively, according to the CDC). Very rarely, seizure disorders, coma, or brain damage has occurred after a DTaP vaccination. Researchers do not know whether these problems were caused by the vaccination or by something else.

> ### Vaccinating Facts
>
> Emil Behring, a German scientist who developed the first diphtheria vaccine in the early 1900s, won the first Nobel Prize in Physiology and Medicine in 1901. He also did research on a tetanus vaccine.

The DTaP vaccine can be given on its own or as a combination vaccine, such as the DTaP and Hib (discussed next) combination vaccine, or a DTaP, Hib, hepatitis B, and polio vaccine (discussed later in this chapter).

> **Health Advisory** _____
>
> An infant having a seizure will often jerk and stiffen. Or, the baby may have few physical signs, and is simply unresponsive or "out of it." Talk to a doctor if a child's behavior or level of consciousness has suddenly changed. Also, never put anything in a child's mouth or hold a child down when he or she is having a seizure. Any seizure lasting more than five minutes needs emergency medical care.

The DTaP vaccine does not provide lifelong immunity. A child will need a booster shot (called the tetanus, diphtheria, and acellular pertussis, or Tdap, shot) around age 11. The booster shot contains a smaller amount of diphtheria and pertussis antigens than the DTaP vaccine. (Adults and seniors also need periodic booster shots to prevent tetanus and diphtheria; you can learn more about this in Chapter 7.)

Who Might Not Get It

Talk to the doctor if brain or nervous system problems develop within a week of a DTaP dose, as it may or may not have triggered underlying neurological problems in the child. Also talk to the doctor if a child has or might have a neurological problem or has had serious side effects after a DTaP shot, such as crying for three or more hours, a fever over 105°F, a seizure, or collapsed after the vaccination.

Haemophilus influenzae type b (Hib)

Haemophilus influenzae type b (Hib) is a contagious bacterial infection, spread by coughing or sneezing, that can cause meningitis (brain and spine infections) and pneumonia (lung infection). Meningitis can cause hearing loss, blindness, or mental retardation, and it can be fatal. Hib can also cause joint problems, blood or bone infections, and breathing problems.

Before the vaccine was used, Hib was a leading cause of bacterial meningitis (the most dangerous type of meningitis) in young children. Each year, about 20,000 U.S. children under five years old became seriously ill from Hib infections. Five percent of the children who developed Hib meningitis died. Today, with Hib vaccination widespread, fewer than 100 children develop Hib infections each year.

The current version of the Hib vaccine was first licensed in the United States in 1985. The Hib vaccine is an inactivated *conjugate vaccine,* meaning it is made by combining a piece of the bacterium's "shell" with a protein (a biological compound) to improve its effectiveness. The protein helps a young child's immune system recognize and respond to the bacterium.

def•i•ni•tion

A **conjugate vaccine** combines disease antigens with a biological compound in order to trigger a strong immune response to the vaccine. Conjugate vaccines are used to create immunity to certain types of bacterial infections in young children, whose immune systems might need help recognizing the bacteria.

Why Now?

Due to its contagious nature, young children between three months and three years old are the most susceptible to a Hib infection. Maternal Hib antibodies are passed on from the mother to a newborn at birth, briefly protecting the infant from infection. The Hib vaccination series is started at two months of age to ensure adequate immunity by the time the mother's antibodies fade.

If an older child or adult has a health problem such as HIV or cancer, a Hib vaccine might be recommended for them. In general, however, the risk of Hib infection is greatest among children under five years old.

What to Expect

The Hib vaccination is given in three or four doses over the course of about a year, depending on the brand. The first dose is given at 2 months of age, the second at 4 months, the third (if necessary per the brand) at 6 months, and a booster dose is given at 12 to 15 months. The Hib vaccine can be combined with other vaccines, such as the hepatitis B vaccine.

The Hib vaccine does not cause serious side effects, but it might cause swelling or soreness at the injection site or a low fever.

Who Might Not Get It

The Hib vaccination should not be given to children under six weeks of age.

Pneumococcal Conjugate Vaccination (PCV7)

Similar to Hib in a number of ways, pneumococcal bacteria are spread by coughing and sneezing. These bacteria can cause pneumonia, meningitis, blood infection, and ear infections. Pneumococcal meningitis in a young child can cause deafness or brain damage, and it can be fatal.

In the past, pneumococcal infections were treated with antibiotics such as penicillin. Yet many strains of pneumococcus bacterium have developed resistance to these antibiotics over time, making the disease much harder to treat. Today, it is possible to decrease pneumococcal infections by vaccinating a young child rather than risking infection and trying to treat it later.

Like the Hib vaccine, the pneumococcal conjugate vaccine (PCV7) for young children is an inactivated conjugate vaccine. A piece of the bacterium's "shell" is linked to a protein carrier in the vaccine that helps trigger a more robust immune system response in a young child. (Older children and adults, whose immune systems are better developed, do not need this carrier to achieve immunity to pneumococcal bacteria.)

The PCV7 was licensed in the United States in 2000, but it does not protect against all the types of bacteria that can cause pneumococcal infections. Instead, it provides immunity against the seven types of bacteria that cause 80 percent of pneumococcal infections in young children. Newer vaccines are currently being developed to provide protection against several more types of pneumococcus bacteria.

Why Now?

Newborn children receive some protection from pneumococcal bacteria from their mother's antibodies. However, as with Hib, the PCV7 series needs to start at two months of age so that the infant has adequate protection by the time the maternal antibodies wear off. Children two years old and under are most likely to get very ill from a pneumococcal infection, which is why it's so important infants get vaccinated. Also, children with a cochlear implant (a medical device used to improve hearing) are at greater risk for pneumococcal infection, so vaccination is especially important for these children.

> **Health Advisory**
>
> Children who attend daycare with other children, as well as African American, Alaska Native, and Native American children, are at increased risk for pneumococcal infections. PCV7 vaccination is especially important for them.

What to Expect

Like the Hib vaccine, the PCV7 is given in a series of four shots at 2 months, 4 months, 6 months, and at 12 to 15 months of age (a booster dose). The PCV7 can be given to an infant as young as six weeks old.

The PCV7 sometimes causes short-term mild side effects such as soreness or redness at the injection site. This is most common after the fourth dose. A child might become fussy, drowsy, have a poor appetite, or develop a fever after one of the doses. In very rare cases, seizures have occurred after PCV vaccination, usually within four days of a dose. It is not known how long the vaccine provides protection—probably for many years. Children five and older are at much lower risk for pneumococcal infections. In general, healthy children and adults (except those 65 and over) do not need further pneumococcal vaccinations.

Who Might Not Get It

In general, all children can safely receive the PCV7 vaccine.

Polio

Polio (also called poliomyelitis) is a viral disease that is spread by contact with stool (such as dirty diapers), coughing, and sneezing. Although the polio virus does not make some people sick, it causes others lifelong muscle paralysis (the inability to move a muscle or limb). If the muscles that help you breathe are paralyzed, it can be fatal. Before effective polio vaccines were developed in the 1950s and 1960s, polio was widespread and greatly feared in the United States. Even today there is no cure for polio.

Vaccinating Facts
Six years before he became a U.S. president, Franklin Delano Roosevelt, who was disabled by polio in 1921, founded the Foundation for Infantile Paralysis (later renamed the March of Dimes) in 1927, a nonprofit polio treatment center. In the mid-1950s, the March of Dimes coordinated the first mass polio vaccination program.

You might have received an oral polio vaccine (OPV) as a child. The OPV was a live, attenuated vaccine that was very effective at creating immunity to polio, and it probably provided lifelong immunity. In very rare cases, however, the OPV caused polio. The OPV vaccine is no longer used in the United States; instead, children are given an inactivated polio vaccine (IPV), which cannot cause polio. The current version of the IPV was licensed in 1990.

Why Now?

Polio is especially dangerous for young children, who are more likely to catch the illness than adults. Maternal antibodies provide temporary protection to a newborn, and then the IPV series is started at two months of age so the child will have adequate protection against polio by the time the maternal antibodies fade.

What to Expect

A child will receive four IPV shots. There is a dose at two months of age (or six weeks at the earliest) and at four months. A third booster dose is given between 6 and 18 months, and the fourth dose (also a booster dose) is given between 4 and 6 years old. If necessary, the IPV can be given on an accelerated schedule, with the first dose at six weeks and the fourth dose given at four and a half months. The IPV is available on its own or as part of a combination vaccine with DTaP and hepatitis B. The IPV can cause soreness at the injection site, but it does not cause any serious side effects. It is not known how long IPV provides protection.

Who Might Not Get It

The IPV contains tiny amounts of the antibiotics called neomycin (found in many topical medications), streptomycin, and polymyxin B. Anyone with a severe allergy to these antibiotics should not receive IPV.

Influenza

Influenza, otherwise known as the flu, is a viral disease spread by coughing and sneezing. It can cause fever, chills, a sore throat, a cough, muscle aches, and other problems. Although most people recover from the flu within a week, it can escalate to pneumonia or other complications. Serious complications from influenza are especially common in very young children and the elderly.

The first influenza vaccine was created in the 1940s, and the current form of the influenza vaccine has been used in the United States since 2001. Now there are two types of influenza vaccines: one is an inactivated vaccine given by injection, and the other is a live, attenuated vaccine given by nasal spray (licensed in 2003). Children under two are given only the inactivated vaccine. Because the viruses that cause influenza are constantly changing, parts of the influenza vaccine are changed yearly to match the viruses predicted to cause influenza in the upcoming flu season. The flu vaccine contains the three types of viruses that researchers believe will cause the greatest number of influenza cases in the upcoming year.

Why Now?

Children two years of age and younger (and the elderly) are more likely to be hospitalized for complications from influenza than people in any other age group, so vaccination is especially important for them. The earliest that children can safely receive a flu shot is six months old.

Children should continue to get a yearly flu shot until they turn 19. Those who live with or care for children under the age of five should also get a flu vaccination (either the live or inactivated vaccine), because the flu can easily be passed on to a child too young to receive a flu shot.

> **Vaccinating Facts**
>
> Yearly influenza rates are usually (but not always) highest in the winter months, especially January. The fall is the best time to get a flu shot.

What to Expect

The flu shot is a one-dose vaccination for adults. But children under the age of nine receiving the vaccine for the first time must receive two doses to ensure immunity. These doses should be given at least one month apart. A child who only received one dose the first year should receive two doses (one month apart) in the next season. After that, a child can receive one yearly dose. Side effects from the vaccination can include soreness at the injection site, aches, fever, and chills for a day or two.

Who Might Not Get It

Children with a severe chicken egg allergy should not receive the flu shot. Cells from chicken eggs are used to make both the live and inactivated vaccines. Also, children under six months of age should not receive a flu shot.

Vaccinations in the First Year of Life by Doctor Visit

Birth	2 Months	4 Months	6 Months
Hepatitis B	Hepatitis B	(Hepatitis B)	Hepatitis B between 6–18 months

Birth	2 Months	4 Months	6 Months
	Rotavirus	Rotavirus	(Rotavirus)
	DTaP	DTaP	DTaP **
	Hib	Hib	(Hib) **
	Pneumococcal conjugate (PCV7)	PCV7	PCV7 **
	Polio (IPV)	Polio (IPV)	Polio (IPV) ** between 6–18 months
			Influenza ***

Note: Vaccine dosages in parentheses might be given if certain brands of vaccine are used.
*** Vaccination series continues into the second year or longer.*
**** The first time a child is vaccinated, he or she needs a second vaccination at least one month later.*

Vaccination Doses Needed in the First Year of Life

Vaccine	Illnesses It Prevents	First-Year Doses
Hepatitis B	Hepatitis B	Birth, 1–2 months, (4 months), 6–18 months
Rotavirus	Rotavirus	2 months, 4 months, (6 months)
DTaP	Diphtheria, tetanus, and acellular pertussis	2 months, 4 months, 6 months **
Hib	*Haemophilus influenzae,* Serotype b infection	2 months, 4 months, (6 months) **
Pneumococcal conjugate	Pneumococcal infection	2 months, 4 months, 6 months **
Polio (IPV)	Polio	2 months, 4 months, 6–18 months **
Influenza	Influenza	6 months ** ***

Note: Vaccine dosages in parentheses might be given if certain brands of vaccine are used.
*** Vaccination series continues into the second year or longer.*
**** The first time a child is vaccinated, he or she needs a second vaccination at least one month later.*

The Least You Need to Know

◆ A child should be vaccinated against nine different diseases in the first year of life.

◆ Many infectious diseases are highly contagious through coughing and sneezing, making vaccination early in life so important.

◆ Most vaccinations are started at two months of age, to build immunity to a disease before maternal antibodies begin to fade.

◆ Some vaccines are combined with others to reduce the number of shots that a child must receive.

5

Vaccinations in the Second Year of Life

In This Chapter

- ◆ The vaccinations continued from the first year to the second year of life
- ◆ The five additional diseases for which children are vaccinated in the second year
- ◆ The effects of these diseases on pregnant women's babies
- ◆ The difference between hepatitis A and hepatitis B

By a child's first birthday, he or she will be fully or partially vaccinated against 9 different diseases. By a child's second birthday, he or she will have received vaccinations against 5 more diseases, providing protection against a total of 14 diseases. All of these vaccinations protect children from sometimes-fatal diseases at an age when they are most vulnerable to catching them. They also protect the adults who care for them.

Continuation from the First Year

For a vaccine to provide protection against a disease, a child needs to receive all the required doses. Some vaccines require doses in both the first and second year of life, and sometimes later as well, to help ensure immunity.

Health Advisory _____

If your child has a life-threatening reaction to a dose of any vaccine, he or she will not receive any more doses of it. If he or she has a life-threatening reaction to a vaccine ingredient, such as a preservative, she might need to avoid other vaccinations as well.

Before your child receives any vaccination, tell your doctor if your child has had any severe reactions to previous vaccinations or is somewhat or very ill with an acute illness. The vaccination might need to be postponed until she is feeling better.

In the second year of life, a child will need additional doses of the following vaccines started in the first year to complete their series:

◆ **Hepatitis B:** Between 6 months and 18 months, a final dose of the vaccine is given to a child whose mother does not have hepatitis B. (A child whose mother *does* have hepatitis B receives the final dose at six months.) This dose completes the vaccination series for hepatitis B.

◆ **Diphtheria, tetanus, and acellular pertussis (DTaP) vaccine:** A fourth dose of the DTaP vaccine is given between 12 months and 18 months of age. This fourth dose should be given at least six months after the third dose. One more dose is given between the ages of four and six to complete the DTaP vaccination series.

◆ *Haemophilus influenzae* **type b (Hib) vaccine:** A final (booster) shot is given at 12 to 15 months of age. This final shot completes the Hib vaccination series.

◆ **Pneumococcal conjugate vaccination (PCV7):** A fourth (booster) shot is given between 12 and 15 months of age. This fourth shot completes the PCV series.

♦ **Inactivated polio vaccine (IPV):** A third dose is given between 6 months and 18 months of age. A fourth (booster) shot is given between ages four and six, which completes the IPV series.

♦ **Influenza vaccine:** A yearly flu shot is given until age 19, preferably in the fall season. A child younger than two years old receives the inactivated vaccine (an injection). A child two years or older can receive the live, attenuated vaccine (a nasal spray).

All the required doses of the rotavirus vaccine are given by the time a child is eight months old, so no further doses are necessary in the second year.

Measles, Mumps, and Rubella (MMR)

Measles, mumps, and rubella are viral diseases, usually spread by coughing and sneezing. Measles and mumps can cause serious health problems for young children, and rubella is a milder disease in children. If a pregnant woman catches rubella, however, the disease can harm her fetus.

The measles virus is so contagious that almost all children were infected with measles in the years before a vaccine was developed. In fact, measles is one of the most contagious infectious diseases that affect humans. Measles has symptoms such as a runny nose, cough, high fever, eye and ear infections, and a rash that spreads from the head downward. A measles infection can also cause pneumonia or, less often, encephalitis (brain inflammation); both can be fatal. Rarely, a person infected with measles can develop a fatal brain inflammation many years after the infection.

Vaccinating Facts
Before the first measles vaccine became available in the 1960s, children aged five to nine were more likely than any other age group to catch measles. In measles outbreaks among unvaccinated people since then, children under five years old have been the most likely to catch it.

The mumps virus is much less contagious than measles, but it has its dangers as well. Mumps causes swollen glands in the neck, fever, and headache, among other symptoms. It can cause meningitis, deafness, and temporary heart inflammation—in rare cases, it is fatal. In adolescents, mumps can make the testicles or ovaries swell and, rarely, can lead to sterility in young men.

Rubella, also called German measles, often causes a facial rash (that gradually moves down the body), swollen lymph glands, and fever in children, although many people who catch rubella show no symptoms of the virus. Rubella can sometimes cause more serious harm such as bleeding problems or brain inflammation. Adults who catch rubella often develop temporary joint pain.

def•i•ni•tion

Congenital rubella syndrome (CRS) causes birth defects in children whose mothers had rubella infections when they were pregnant. CRS symptoms can include mental retardation or problems with vision and hearing.

If a pregnant woman catches rubella from a child or an adult, the virus is likely to cause a miscarriage or birth defects, especially if she catches rubella in the first trimester. Although it is rare in the United States, *congenital rubella syndrome* (*CRS*), caused by a pregnant woman's rubella infection, can cause birth defects such as visual impairment, deafness, and mental retardation. Children born with CRS are more likely to develop diabetes, brain disease, or autism when they get older. Because rubella is so dangerous during pregnancy, children are vaccinated against rubella to prevent them from spreading the virus to adults and to protect them from the virus when they reach adulthood.

Vaccinating Facts

You may have heard about studies that link the MMR vaccine to autism. In children who are later diagnosed with autism, parents often begin to notice symptoms of autism around the time their children receive their MMR vaccination. Recent studies, however, have found no link between the MMR vaccination and autism. Learn more about this issue in Chapter 12.

The measles, mumps, and rubella (MMR) vaccine, licensed in 1971, is a live, attenuated vaccine. In the past, children received one dose of

MMR, which created immunity to measles for 95 percent of children. Researchers found that a second dose, however, improves measles immunity levels up to about 99 percent of vaccinated children. The two-dose MMR vaccine creates immunity to mumps and rubella in 95 percent of children vaccinated. This second dose of MMR is primarily given to ensure the maximum immunity levels possible to measles. The second dose also helps provide immunity to children who may have missed the first dose.

Vaccinating Facts

The Pan American Health Organization (PAHO) is working to eliminate congenital rubella syndrome (CRS) in the Caribbean and North, Central, and South America by 2010. To reach this goal, PAHO is supporting MMR vaccinations in the Americas and collecting data on rubella outbreaks. Congenital rubella syndrome was eliminated in the United States in 2005 through vaccination, and rubella cases in the Americas decreased 98 percent from 1998 to 2006. Despite rubella outbreaks in Brazil, Argentina, and Chile in 2007, PAHO will most likely meet its 2010 goal.

Why Now?

Because measles in particular is so contagious, the MMR vaccine is given to young children as early as possible. If mothers caught these viruses as children or were vaccinated against measles, mumps, and rubella, their newborn infants receive some protection from the maternal antibodies in their blood. The MMR vaccine, like most live vaccines, is usually not given to children less than a year old because maternal antibodies in the child's blood are present and could make the vaccine less effective.

What to Expect

Children should receive the first dose of the MMR vaccine between 12 and 15 months of age. They should receive the second dose between four and six years of age, ideally before they start kindergarten and have greater exposure to other children and infectious diseases. If necessary, the second dose can be given as soon as four weeks after the first dose.

The doctor might do this if a child is immunized later than recommended, or to help ensure immunity if there is a measles, mumps, or rubella outbreak in the area.

Health Advisory

What do you do if a child less than a year old is exposed to measles? A child six months old or older can receive the MMR vaccination or a single measles vaccination, if necessary, although maternal antibodies could make the vaccines less effective. The child must receive the MMR vaccination within three days of exposure to measles, during the incubation period of the virus, to be protected against it. When he or she reaches 12 months old, the MMR vaccine should be received on the standard schedule. A child younger than six months old is probably adequately protected from measles by maternal antibodies.

After vaccination, a child might feel sore or be swollen at the injection site, develop a mild rash, or have temporarily swollen glands or lymph nodes. About one to two weeks after vaccination, some children develop a fever of 103°F or higher for a day or two. A quarter of all teens and adults develop temporary pain in their joints within a few weeks of MMR vaccination, but this problem is rare in children. Very rarely, a child has a seizure triggered by a post-vaccination fever, or develops a temporary bleeding disorder after MMR vaccination.

The MMR vaccine is sometimes combined with the varicella (chickenpox) vaccine (discussed next) to reduce the number of shots a child needs. This combination is called the measles, mumps, rubella, and varicella (MMRV) vaccine, and it was available for children under 13 years old. The MMRV was taken off the market for further study because it might increase the risk of fever seizures after vaccination. The vaccine might be available again in the future, however.

The MMR vaccine is believed to provide lifelong immunity to measles, mumps, and rubella, but mumps immunity might not be lifelong.

Who Might Not Get It

If a child has cancer, has a disease that suppresses the immune system, or is receiving treatments that suppress the immune system, a doctor should be consulted about whether the child should receive the MMR vaccination. Also, consult a doctor if a child has received blood products (such as a blood transfusion) or has had any bleeding disorders, because the vaccination may need to be postponed or skipped for these children.

The MMR vaccine contains gelatin, sorbitol, and the antibiotic neomycin. If a child is severely allergic to any of these substances, he or she might not receive the vaccine. The MMR vaccination also contains a small amount of chicken egg materials, but it is still considered safe for children with severe egg allergies.

Varicella (Chickenpox)

As a child, you probably caught chickenpox, recovered from it, and then developed immunity to the varicella zoster virus that causes chickenpox. Chickenpox, which is spread through the air and by physical contact with an infected person, causes (as you may remember) an itchy rash of blisters, fever, and fatigue. Sometimes the rash can leave permanent scars.

Chickenpox infections are usually mild in children. But, the virus can cause complications such as pneumonia or encephalitis in some children. The skin rash from chickenpox can become infected with dangerous bacteria as well, creating a life-threatening infection. The chickenpox vaccine was developed to protect children from its complications and to prevent the spread of the disease.

> **Vaccinating Facts**
>
> Chickenpox is not a disease spread by chickens. Instead, experts believe that the name of the disease is derived from the Latin word *cicer,* meaning "chickpea." Chickenpox blisters look like chickpeas.

If adolescents or adults catch chickenpox, they can become seriously ill. They are far more likely than children to be hospitalized or die from chickenpox. If a pregnant woman catches chickenpox around her first trimester of pregnancy, her child has a 2 percent chance of developing birth defects, such as low birth weight, shortened limbs, and scarring.

After a person recovers from chickenpox, the virus remains in the body for life. It sometimes reactivates in middle age or later (although it can occur earlier) in the form of shingles (or herpes zoster), which causes a rash and nerve pain. About 20 percent of people will develop shingles at some time in their life. If you are vaccinated against chickenpox as a child, shingles is less likely to develop, and if it occurs it is usually fairly mild. For adults who are too old to have received the chickenpox vaccination as children, the herpes zoster vaccine can help prevent shingles. You can learn more about that vaccine in Chapter 7.

Health Advisory

Parents are more likely to refuse the MMR or varicella (chickenpox) vaccine for their children than any other childhood vaccines, according to surveys of pediatricians done by the American Academy of Pediatrics. Some parents believe that these vaccines can harm their children, or that they are unnecessary for healthy children. Although most chickenpox infections are mild, chickenpox sometimes causes serious or fatal complications in children. These complications tend to occur among children who were healthy before they caught the virus.

The chickenpox vaccine is a live, attenuated vaccine. It was licensed for use in the United States in 1995. The vaccine was licensed for use earlier in Japan and Korea in 1988, so it has been studied for over 20 years.

Why Now?

Like the measles virus, the chickenpox virus is quite contagious. As a result, children are more likely to catch chickenpox when they are around other children. For this reason, the doses of the chickenpox vaccine are given to children around the time they might enter daycare and elementary school.

The timing of the first vaccine dose, at 12 to 15 months of age, is especially important. Children ages one to four are more likely to catch chickenpox than people in most other age groups. Because it is a live vaccine, the chickenpox vaccine is less effective on children less than 12 months old due to the maternal antibodies in their blood.

What to Expect

The chickenpox vaccination schedule is similar to the MMR schedule. A child receives the first dose at 12 to 15 months of age, and the second dose at 4 to 6 years of age. If needed, the second dose can be given as early as three months after the first dose.

A second dose of the chickenpox vaccine is recommended because sometimes a child can have a "breakthrough" case of chickenpox after the first dose. Although these infections are milder than what an unvaccinated child would catch, a child with a breakthrough infection can pass it on to others. The second dose helps prevent these infections when a child is in elementary school and likely to be in close contact with many other children.

Sometimes, the chickenpox vaccine is combined with the MMR vaccine into an MMRV vaccine. Because it's best not to give the second chickenpox vaccine sooner than three months after the first dose, the two MMRV doses should be administered at least three months apart. The MMRV vaccine should be given only to children 12 years old and younger.

Health Advisory

If your child receives the chickenpox vaccination separately from the MMR vaccination, he should receive both vaccinations on the same day or receive the chickenpox vaccination at least 30 days after the MMR vaccination. If he receives the chickenpox vaccination from 1 to 29 days after the MMR vaccination, the chickenpox vaccination might not be as effective.

Side effects occur most often after the first dose of the chickenpox vaccine. They are also more likely after an MMRV vaccination. After the chickenpox vaccination, a child might be sore or swollen at the injection site. Some children develop a fever within about a month of vaccination (often this fever is not caused by the vaccination), and some develop a rash within about three weeks. Rarely, a fever causes a seizure or a child develops pneumonia after the vaccination. Serious complications (such as brain problems) after a chickenpox vaccination are extremely rare and difficult to link to the vaccination.

The chickenpox vaccine is thought to provide lifelong immunity to the varicella virus.

Who Might Not Get It

Children with a severe allergy to gelatin or the antibiotic neomycin might need to skip the chickenpox vaccine. Consult a doctor if a child has received blood products, such as a blood transfusion, because the vaccination might need to be postponed. Also, consult a doctor if a child has cancer or a chronic illness that suppresses the immune system, or if the child is receiving medical treatments that suppress the immune system.

Hepatitis A

Most young children who catch the hepatitis A virus exhibit no symptoms of the disease. Adults can become very ill, however, if they catch it from children. Hepatitis A is very contagious, and it is usually spread through contact with infected stool. For example, an adult might catch the virus by not properly washing his or her hands after changing the diaper of a baby who has hepatitis A. It can also be spread through contaminated food or water.

The hepatitis A virus (like the hepatitis B virus) affects your liver, causing jaundice (yellowing of eyes and skin), fever, nausea, diarrhea, stomach pains, and other problems. On average, an adult who has hepatitis A misses about a month of work, and often must be hospitalized. Hepatitis A usually goes away on its own after about two months, but it can last as long as six months. In rare cases, hepatitis A can be fatal.

Because the virus is common in many parts of the world—including Central America, Africa, and Asia—many travelers need to be vaccinated against the virus before they go abroad. (More on this and other vaccines recommended for travel in Chapter 10.) Certain other groups are at greater risk for catching hepatitis A as well, including people living with someone with hepatitis A and men who have sex with other men. About half of the people who catch hepatitis A, however, don't have any of these risk factors and don't know how they caught it.

Brain Booster _____

Hepatitis A and hepatitis B have similar names and symptoms, but they have distinct differences.

♦ Hepatitis A is always an acute (short-term) illness, but hepatitis B can be an acute or chronic (long-term) illness.

♦ Hepatitis A is usually spread by contact with infected stool, but hepatitis B is usually spread by contact with infected bodily fluids (such as blood).

♦ Hepatitis A can be transmitted through food and drink, but hepatitis B cannot.

♦ A pregnant woman infected with hepatitis A is unlikely to pass it on to her baby, but she is likely to pass on hepatitis B.

The hepatitis A vaccine is an inactivated vaccine created from the whole virus, not part of it. The vaccine was licensed in 1995.

Why Now?

Although they usually don't exhibit symptoms, young children often pass on hepatitis A to people in their household, who in turn become very ill. Children are vaccinated against the disease as soon as possible to protect the adults and other children around them.

Unlike the hepatitis B virus, which an infected mother can pass on to her baby during birth, the hepatitis A virus is usually not passed on during birth. Yet an infected mother with hepatitis A or anyone else with hepatitis A can pass the virus on to the newborn through close contact with the child.

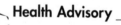 **Health Advisory** _____

Hepatitis A vaccination is especially important for children who are Alaska Natives or Native American. People in these ethnic groups are at greater risk for hepatitis A infection.

What to Expect

Children are given two doses of a special children's formulation of the hepatitis A vaccine to ensure immunity. They receive the first dose at

12 months of age or older, when any maternal antibodies to hepatitis A have faded away. They receive the second (booster) dose 6 to 12 months after the first dose (for one type of vaccine), or 6 to 18 months after the first dose (for the other type of vaccine). Researchers have found that these two doses provide about 100 percent protection against hepatitis A among children.

Some children feel sore at the injection site or develop a headache after the vaccination. A child might briefly lose his or her appetite after the vaccination, and it can also cause temporary flulike symptoms such as fatigue and a low fever. These mild side effects usually go away a day or two after the shot.

Because the vaccine has been available only since the mid-1990s, it is unknown whether the immunity it creates is lifelong. Researchers believe, though, that the vaccine provides at least 20 years of immunity to hepatitis A.

Who Might Not Get It

Children with a severe allergy to alum (a substance used to boost the effectiveness of the vaccine) or 2-phenoxyethanol (a vaccine preservative) may need to skip getting the vaccine. Children allergic to 2-phenoxyethanol can receive a hepatitis A vaccine that does not contain this ingredient. Adequate hand washing can help protect children who cannot receive the vaccination from hepatitis A and other infectious diseases.

Vaccinations in the Second Year of Life by Doctor Visit

Vaccination	Doctor Visit
Hepatitis B	6 to 18 months old
DTaP	15 to 18 months old **
Hib	12 to 15 months
Pneumococcal (PCV)	12 to 15 months
Polio (IPV)	6 to 18 months **
Influenza	Once a year, preferably in the fall ** ***
MMR or MMRV	12 to 15 months **

Vaccination	Doctor Visit
Varicella (chickenpox)	12 to 15 months **
Hepatitis A	12 and 18–24 months (or 18–30 months) **

Note: Vaccine dosages in parentheses might be given if certain brands of vaccine are used.
** Vaccination series might continue into the third year or longer.
*** The first time a child is vaccinated, he or she needs a second vaccination at least one month later.

Vaccination Doses Needed in the Second Year of Life

Vaccine	Illnesses It Prevents	Second-Year Doses
Hepatitis B	Hepatitis B	Final dose at 6–18 months
DTaP	Diphtheria, tetanus, pertussis	One dose at 15–18 months **
Hib	*Haemophilus influenzae* type b	Final dose at 12–15 months
Pneumococcal type b	Pneumococcal infections	Final dose at 12–15 months
Polio (IPV)	Polio	One dose at 6–18 months **
Influenza	Influenza	One dose in the fall ** ***
MMR or MMRV	Measles, mumps, rubella, varicella	One dose at 12–15 months **
Varicella	Chickenpox	One dose at 12–15 months **
Hepatitis A	Hepatitis A infection	Two doses, at 12 months and at 18–24 months (or 18–30 months) **

Note: Vaccine dosages in parentheses might be given if certain brands of vaccine are used.
** Vaccination series might continue into the third year or longer.
*** The first time a child is vaccinated, he or she needs a second vaccination at least one month later.

The Least You Need to Know

◆ Children receive the MMR, varicella, and hepatitis A vaccinations in their second year of life.

◆ A measles vaccination is important because it is one of the most infectious diseases in people.

◆ Rubella and chickenpox infections can be dangerous to a pregnant woman's baby.

◆ Hepatitis A is very contagious and often has no symptoms in infected children.

Chapter 6

For Ages 2 to 18 Years

In This Chapter

- Remaining doses a child needs to complete childhood vaccinations series
- What to do if a vaccination is missed
- The importance of the yearly influenza vaccine
- The Tdap booster, HPV for girls, and meningococcal vaccines

After a flurry of vaccinations during the first and second years, the number of recommended vaccinations slows down throughout the rest of childhood. By age six, children will have received the remaining doses of many vaccination series that they began at less than two years of age. At age 11 to 12, they receive a few more vaccinations to complete all their recommended childhood vaccinations. If they missed any vaccinations, they can also receive catch-up doses later in childhood or in adolescence.

From Ages Two to Six

If a child is healthy and receives the recommended vaccinations on schedule in the first and second years of life, he or she will not be vaccinated against any new diseases until age 11. Instead, in these years, a child will receive the final doses of many childhood vaccination series that were already started. When a child is between ages four and six years old, he or she will receive ...

- The fifth and final dose of the diphtheria, tetanus, and acellular pertussis (DTaP) vaccine.

- The fourth and final dose of the inactivated polio (IPV) vaccine.

- The second and final dose of the measles, mumps, and rubella (MMR) vaccine.

- The second and final dose of the varicella (chickenpox) vaccine.

If a child did not receive a standard hepatitis A vaccination at a younger age (because the recommended age for hepatitis A vaccination has changed in recent years), he or she might receive one between ages two and six. A child with chronic conditions or other health problems might receive extra vaccinations between ages two and six (learn more about these in Chapter 8).

Catch-Up Vaccinations

If a child missed some or all of the recommended vaccinations when he or she was less than two years old, the child can receive catch-up childhood vaccinations. These can be given on their own or as a combination vaccination that includes other vaccines. For example, one catch-up combination vaccination includes the hepatitis B, DTaP, and IPV vaccines.

Brain Booster

If your child missed some vaccinations, the CDC's Catch-Up Immunization Scheduler for children six and under can help you learn what vaccinations he or she needs and when. It is available on the CDC website at www.cdc.gov/print.do?url=http://www.cdc.gov/vaccines/recs/scheduler/catchup.htm. Enter your child's birth date and the dates and doses of vaccinations received to date to find out when any catch-up vaccinations should be scheduled.

If necessary, the catch-up vaccination recommendations for children four months to six years of age are as follows:

Catch-Up Vaccines up to Age 6

Vaccine	Minimum Time from Dose 1 to 2	Minimum Time from Dose 2 to 3	Minimum Time from Dose 3 to 4	Minimum Time from Dose 4 to 5	Notes
Hepatitis B	4 weeks	8 weeks			The first and last doses should be at least 4 months apart.
Rotavirus	4 weeks	4 weeks			It may require either two or three doses. This should not be given to children 8 months or older, and the series should not be started in infants aged 15 weeks or older.
Diphtheria, tetanus, and acellular pertussis (DTaP)	4 weeks	4 weeks	6 months	6 months	If a child received the fourth dose at age 4 or older, the fifth dose is not needed.

continues

Catch-Up Vaccines up to Age 6 (continued)

Vaccine	Minimum Time from Dose 1 to 2	Minimum Time from Dose 2 to 3	Minimum Time from Dose 3 to 4	Minimum Time from Dose 4 to 5	Notes
Hib	4 to 8 weeks, depending on age and vaccination record	4 to 8 weeks, depending on age and vaccination record	8 weeks (fourth dose only required in certain circumstances)		Not usually given to children 5 years or older.
Pneumococcal	4 to 8 weeks, depending on age and vaccination record	4 to 8 weeks, depending on age	8 weeks		A child might only need two or three doses, depending on age, vaccination record, and health.
Inactivated polio (IPV)	4 weeks	4 weeks	4 weeks		A child might only need three doses, depending on age and vaccination record.
Measles, mumps, and rubella (MMR)	4 weeks				If possible, a child should receive the second dose at 4 to 6 years.

Vaccine	Minimum Time from Dose 1 to 2	Minimum Time from Dose 2 to 3	Minimum Time from Dose 3 to 4	Minimum Time from Dose 4 to 5	Notes
Varicella (chickenpox)	3 months is best; 4 weeks is okay if a child is 12 months or older				If possible, a child should receive the second dose at 4 to 6 years.
Hepatitis A	6 months				Recommended for children over 12 months if hepatitis A is a problem in the area.

A child can also receive many catch-up vaccinations between ages 7 and 18. They are as follows:

Catch-Up Vaccines Ages 7–18

Vaccine	Minimum time from Dose 1 to 2	Minimum time from Dose 2 to 3	Minimum time from Dose 3 to 4	Notes
Hepatitis B	4 weeks	8 weeks		The third dose should be given at least 4 months after the first dose.
Tetanus, diphtheria, and pertussis (Td/Tdap)	4 weeks	4 weeks or 6 months, depending on when/if a child received previous DTaP or Tdap doses	6 months, if a child received a DTaP vaccination as an infant	If a child received the fourth dose at age 4 or older, the fifth dose is not needed. Tdap may be substituted for one dose of Td in children ages 10–18.
Inactivated polio (IPV)	4 weeks	4 weeks	4 weeks	A child might only need three doses of polio vaccine, depending on age and vaccination record.

Vaccine	Minimum time from Dose 1 to 2	Minimum time from Dose 2 to 3	Minimum time from Dose 3 to 4	Notes
Measles, mumps, and rubella (MMR)	4 weeks			
Varicella (chickenpox)	3 months is best; 4 weeks is okay, especially in ages 13 and older			
Hepatitis A	6 months			
Human papillomavirus (HPV)	4 weeks	12 weeks		The third dose should be given at least 6 months after the first dose.

Health Advisory

Healthy children can usually receive all their vaccinations on the recommended schedule. If your child has a life-threatening reaction to a
dose of a vaccine, however, he or she will not receive more doses of it.
If he or she has a life-threatening reaction to a vaccine ingredient, such
as a preservative, he or she might need to avoid other vaccinations as
well.

Before your child receives a vaccination, be sure to tell your doctor if
your child has had any severe reactions to previous vaccinations or is
somewhat or very ill with an acute (short-term) illness. The vaccination
might need to be postponed until he or she is feeling better.

Influenza

A child will continue to receive a routine yearly influenza vaccination
until he or she is 18 years old. Children under two years old can receive
only the inactivated influenza vaccine, which is given by injection.
Children two years old and older, however, can receive either the inactivated, injected influenza vaccine or the live, attenuated influenza vaccine (LAIV). The LAIV, licensed for use in the United States in 2003,
is given by nasal spray.

Why Now?

The flu is contagious, and it easily gets passed around in households and
daycare settings. Both children and adults should receive a yearly flu
shot to prevent infection. Especially while a child is under five years old,
the household members should also get a yearly influenza vaccination to
protect the child. In most cases, household members can receive either
the live or inactivated influenza vaccine, depending on their health.

For the child, getting the inactivated vaccine is the best if ...

♦ He or she has a chronic condition such as asthma, heart disease,
diabetes, or a seizure disorder.

♦ He or she is receiving medical treatments that weaken the immune
system, or has an illness that weakens the immune system.

♦ He or she is receiving aspirin therapy.

In general, all other children can receive LAIV, thereby avoiding another injection.

Brain Booster

The viruses that cause influenza change from year to year, yet many people do not get their yearly recommended flu shot. As a result, influenza outbreaks are far more common in the United States than other vaccine-preventable diseases. Influenza infections can cause pneumonia and other serious problems, leading to over 200,000 hospitalizations and about 36,000 deaths each year. Young children and the elderly are most likely to become seriously ill from influenza, making vaccination especially important for these groups.

What to Expect

The first time a child under nine years old receives either the inactivated or the live influenza vaccine, he or she should get two doses of it, with the second dose given at least four weeks after the first dose. Ideally, a child should receive the first dose in September or October so the two doses are completed before the winter months, when influenza is most common. After that, a child can receive just one dose of either vaccine each year (between September and November, if possible).

A child can receive other live vaccines, such as the varicella (chickenpox) vaccine, on the same day as the LAIV. If another live vaccine is not given on the same day as the LAIV, however, a child should not receive the other live vaccine for at least a month. A live vaccine given too soon after the LAIV might prevent the LAIV from working effectively. The live influenza vaccine can cause mild, short-term side effects such as a runny nose, fever, and wheezing.

Who Might Not Get It

Consult a doctor if a child has a severe egg allergy because he or she might not be able to have either influenza vaccination. Children with severe allergies to MSG, gelatin, arginine (an amino acid sometimes used to treat medical problems), or the antibiotic gentamicin should not receive the LAIV. If a child has a serious nasal problem, he or she might not be able to receive the LAIV. Also consult a doctor if a child has had Guillain-Barré Syndrome (GBS). This rare nervous system problem, which can cause temporary paralysis or (more rarely) death, was linked to an influenza vaccine that was distributed in 1976. A history of GBS might make a child more susceptible to it after either type of influenza vaccination. Sometimes GBS occurs after other vaccinations as well. This happens so rarely, however, that it is often difficult for researchers to know whether the vaccination caused it.

Tetanus, Diphtheria, and Acellular Pertussis (Tdap)

Not to be confused with DTaP, the tetanus, diphtheria, and acellular pertussis (Tdap) vaccination is something a little bit different, but it is still in the same family. Tdap is a booster dose of the DTaP vaccination a child received between two months and six years of age.

Vaccinating Facts

Different letters are capitalized in the DTaP (diphtheria, tetanus, and acellular pertussis) and Tdap (tetanus, diphtheria, and acellular pertussis) acronyms to show different levels of antigen in these vaccines. Capitalization indicates a greater amount of antigen in the vaccine than a lowercase letter. Therefore, the DTaP vaccine has a higher amount of diphtheria (D) toxoid and pertussis (P) antigen than the Tdap booster.

Why Now?

Although children receive vaccinations against diphtheria, tetanus, and pertussis (the DTaP vaccination discussed in the previous chapter) when they are younger, this immunity wears off over time. Because the DTaP vaccination tends to cause more side effects in children over seven years old than those under seven, the Tdap vaccination was created and licensed in 2005. This vaccine contains smaller amounts of diphtheria and pertussis antigens—that's why the "d" and "p" are lowercase—which decreases the chances of causing side effects in older children and adults.

What to Expect

Older children who have completed their DTaP vaccinations should get one dose of Tdap when they are 11 or 12 years old. If necessary, older children can get one of the two available brands of Tdap vaccines when they are as young as 10 years old. The other brand is only approved for children 11 and older.

Before 2005 and the Tdap vaccination, older children received a tetanus and diphtheria (Td) booster vaccination. Because pertussis can be dangerous for older children, and they can also pass it on to younger children, Tdap is now the standard booster vaccination for older children, and a child should get one dose of Tdap if he or she has not yet received it. If a child received a Td vaccination in the past, it's best to wait five years before getting a Tdap vaccination, unless he or she is at increased risk for catching pertussis. If the Tdap vaccination is given too close to the Td vaccination, a child might have a more severe reaction to the vaccine.

Common side effects from the Tdap vaccination in older children include pain or swelling at the injection site, headache, fatigue, and nausea. Most older children will have one or more of these side effects after vaccination. Fever occurs less often after vaccination. Extremely rarely, an older child might feel severe pain or swelling at the injection site.

Who Might Not Get It

If a child had seizures or went into a coma within a week of a childhood DTaP vaccination, he or she might not receive a Tdap vaccination. Consult a doctor if a child has a severe latex allergy or if a child has a nervous system disorder or epilepsy, has had Guillain-Barré syndrome (GBS), or has had severe pain or swelling after receiving a previous dose of DTaP, Td, or a related vaccine.

Human Papillomavirus (HPV)

There are about 40 different types of human papillomavirus (HPV) viruses that are frequently spread by sexual contact. These viruses often cause mild infections that cause no symptoms and go away on their own. Sexually transmitted HPV viruses are extremely common. By age 50, researchers estimate that about 80 percent of sexually active women will have had an HPV infection.

Although most HPV infections are harmless, a few of the HPV viruses can cause chronic infections that lead to cancers such as cervical, anal, and throat cancer. Some of the HPV viruses can also cause genital warts, and HPV infections can be harmful in pregnant women as well. A pregnant woman infected with HPV can pass it on to her newborn during birth, which can lead to a sometimes-fatal throat problem in the child.

The HPV vaccine can prevent infection from four of the most damaging HPV viruses. These four viruses cause about 70 percent of all cervical cancers, a very common cancer in women, and about 90 percent of all genital warts. However, a woman who has received the HPV vaccine might still develop cervical cancer or genital warts if she becomes chronically infected with one of the other HPV viruses not included in the vaccine. But, the vaccine does greatly reduce her chances of developing these diseases.

The HPV vaccine is an inactivated vaccine, first licensed in the United States in 2006. Another HPV vaccine is under development and may be approved at the end of 2009.

Why Now?

Girls are vaccinated with the HPV vaccine at 11 or 12 years old to create immune system protection against HPV infection, ideally before they become sexually active. If necessary, they can be vaccinated as young as nine years old. If they are vaccinated after they become infected with one of the viruses in the HPV vaccine, the vaccine cannot prevent that HPV infection.

The HPV vaccine can be received at a later age as well, because the HPV vaccine is approved for young women up to age 26. It provides the best protection if received before becoming sexually active.

Health Advisory

Because of its link to cervical cancer, HPV vaccine researchers initially focused on girls and women. However, sexually active men can spread HPV viruses, too. Like women, men can also develop genital warts and certain cancers from HPV infections. The effect of the HPV vaccine on boys and men is currently being studied. To help protect both women and men from infection, the HPV vaccine will probably be recommended for preteen boys in the near future.

Some parents object to the HPV vaccine because it is often given to girls at a young age. They believe that the vaccine might encourage girls to become sexually active earlier. Because of these concerns, few states currently require the HPV vaccine in order for girls to attend school. Other vaccines, such as the MMR and DTaP vaccines, are required for school entry in most states. Learn more about vaccination requirements and exemptions later in Chapter 13.

What to Expect

Girls receive three doses of the vaccine, usually when they are 11 or 12 years old, over a period of six months. The vaccinations should follow this dosing schedule:

◆ The second dose is usually given two months after the first dose, but it can be given as soon as four weeks after the first dose.

◆ The third dose is usually given 4 months after the second dose, but it can be given as soon as 12 weeks after the second dose.

The second and third doses should not *both* be given early. The third dose should be given at least six months after the first dose.

Common side effects from the HPV vaccine include pain, swelling, or itching at the injection site, and fever. There are no known severe side effects from the vaccine. Because the HPV vaccine is relatively new, researchers do not yet know how long it provides immunity against HPV infections.

Brain Booster

The HPV vaccine is the most expensive childhood vaccine, costing about $390 for three doses when purchased by private health-care providers, according to the CDC's 2009 Vaccine Price List. By comparison, some other childhood vaccines are much cheaper, such as the five-dose DTaP vaccine (about $105 to $115 for all the doses) and the four-dose Hib vaccine (about $92 for all the doses). Some health insurers and federal programs cover the cost of the vaccine and negotiate lower prices. If your insurer does not cover this cost, you might need to pay for the vaccine yourself.

Who Might Not Get It

If a girl or young woman has a life-threatening allergy to yeast, she should not receive the HPV vaccine. The HPV vaccine is made using yeast cells.

Meningococcal Vaccination

The bacteria *Neisseria meningitidis*, which cause meningococcal infections, can live in your upper airway without causing any problems. But if they cross a mucous membrane (a physical barrier of the immune system) and enter the bloodstream, they can infect the lining of the brain (called meningitis), infect the blood (called sepsis), or cause other problems such as pneumonia. Having certain immune problems can make meningococcal infections more likely.

Meningitis, which can be fatal, causes symptoms such as headache, stiff neck, and a high fever. Sepsis, which is less common than meningitis but more often fatal in children, has symptoms such as a fever and coma. Meningococcal infections can lead to permanent health problems, including deafness, nervous system problems, mental retardation, or loss of a limb due to circulation problems.

Bacterial meningitis and sepsis often develop extremely quickly. For example, a child can become infected and die of sepsis in less than a day. Although antibiotics like penicillin can be used to treat these infections, the infection is sometimes too aggressive to treat effectively by the time it is diagnosed. That is why vaccination is recommended to prevent meningococcal disease.

Meningococcal bacteria are spread through physical contact with oral secretions, such as through kissing or sharing food. An infected person can spread the bacteria through sneezing, sending oral droplets into the air that others could breathe. Also, living with someone with a meningococcal infection puts a person at a higher than average risk of catching the infection. Outbreaks are more common when people are in close quarters for several hours at a time, such as in a dormitory or child care center.

In the 1970s, a meningococcal polysaccharide vaccine (MPSV4) was developed to prevent meningococcal infections. It is still used today to vaccinate older adults, but the structure of the vaccine does not create immunity in young children. A newer meningococcal conjugate vaccine (MCV4), licensed in 2005, is considered more effective in young children, adolescents, and adults 55 or younger. MCV4 is also better at preventing the bacteria from spreading from person to person than MPSV4. Today, a child will most likely receive the newer MCV4. MCV4 is an inactivated vaccine that combines pieces of the meningococcal bacteria with pieces of diphtheria toxoid (killed diphtheria toxins). This combination helps improve a body's immune response to the meningococcal bacterium.

The MCV4 vaccine protects against four of the common types of bacteria that cause meningococcal disease. It does not provide protection against all the types of bacteria that could cause meningococcal disease, but it protects from some of the most common ones in the United States.

Why Now?

Meningococcal infections are most common in children less than 2 years old, people who have a chronic medical problem, and people ages 15 to 24. Most children are vaccinated against meningococcal disease at 11 or 12 years old, before their risk of catching the disease increases. Adolescents can also be vaccinated with MCV4 up to age 18. Vaccination is important if a child will be living in a crowded area where the disease can spread rapidly, such as a college dormitory. In fact, to prevent outbreaks, some colleges and universities require a meningococcal vaccination before the start of school.

If a young child is at special risk for infection (because she has a chronic disease, for example), he or she will receive an MCV4 as early as age two, but this is not a standard vaccination in young children. The MCV4 vaccine does not work well on children under two years old.

What to Expect

A child will receive one dose of MCV4 at age 11 or 12. Sometimes a child 10 or younger will receive a dose of MCV4 if he or she is at high risk of catching meningococcal disease.

Pain or redness at the injection site, lasting for a day or two, is a common MCV4 side effect. A preteen might also develop a fever, headache, and other mild problems after the vaccination, usually within a week of the vaccination. In very rare cases, people have developed Guillain-Barré syndrome (GBS) after MCV4 vaccination. Researchers do not know whether these cases of GBS were caused by the vaccination. Vaccination with MCV4 is believed to provide protection for several years, but researchers are still studying how long MCV4 immunity lasts.

Who Might Not Get It

Consult a doctor if a child has a severe latex allergy, if he or she has had a severe response to the diphtheria toxoid in previous vaccinations (such as the DTaP or Tdap), or if he or she has ever had GBS. In these cases, a child might not be able to receive a meningococcal vaccine.

Vaccinations for Ages 2 to 18 Years

Age	Vaccination
2–18	Influenza (inactivated or LAIV) each fall. *
4–6	DTaP vaccine (diphtheria, tetanus, and acellular pertussis vaccine), one final dose.
	IPV vaccine (inactivated polio vaccine), one final dose.

Age	Vaccination
	MMR or MMRV vaccine (measles, mumps, and rubella, +/-varicella vaccine), one final dose.
	Varicella (chickenpox vaccine), one final dose.
11–12	Tdap vaccine (tetanus, diphtheria, and acellular pertussis booster), one dose (one brand can be given as young as 10 years old).
	HPV vaccine (human papillomavirus vaccine), three doses for girls (can be given as young as 9 years old). The second HPV dose is usually given two months after the first dose, and the third dose is given at least six months after the first dose.
	Meningococcal vaccine (MCV4), one dose (can be given at a younger age to high-risk children).

* *The first time a child is vaccinated, he or she needs a second vaccination at least one month later.*

The Least You Need to Know

◆ All of the doses of most childhood vaccinations are completed by age six.

◆ If a vaccination series or dose is missed, there are special catch-up vaccination schedules for certain ages.

◆ A child should continue to receive a yearly influenza vaccination until the age of 18.

◆ Adolescent girls and young women can be vaccinated with HPV to protect them from certain cancers.

◆ Meningococcal infections are contagious among children.

Chapter 7

Staying Healthy Throughout Adulthood

In This Chapter

- ◆ Vaccinations all adults should have
- ◆ Special vaccines for young adults and seniors
- ◆ Managing vaccines when there are health problems
- ◆ Recommendations for young women and pregnant women
- ◆ Recommendations for people with certain occupations and lifestyles

Adults may think they don't need any vaccinations, or may be confused about what vaccinations are needed in adulthood. Depending on age, adults may still be well-protected by their childhood vaccinations—but that doesn't mean they are protected as much as they could be. In this chapter, we'll explore vaccinations that are a good idea to get in adulthood and in certain circumstances.

Are We Done Yet?

You might be wondering why adults would need any more vaccinations, assuming they have received all the recommended childhood vaccinations. Aren't we done with all these shots?

While researchers believe that many childhood vaccinations provide long-term immunity to a disease or group of diseases, there often is not enough data to predict exactly how long immunity lasts. Some childhood vaccines are known to provide immunity for only 5 or 10 years. Many vaccines, especially inactivated vaccines, provide less effective protection as time goes by, so adults may need a booster dose of some childhood vaccinations to stay protected against certain diseases.

 Brain Booster

> To learn what vaccinations you need as an adult, take the Centers for Disease Control and Prevention's (CDC) interactive Adolescent and Adult Vaccine Quiz available online at www2.cdc.gov/nip/adultImmSched/. When you finish the quiz, you will be given vaccination recommendations to discuss with your doctor.

Many adults are too old to have received certain childhood vaccinations because they weren't available when they were younger. Many currently recommended vaccines for children or adolescents were licensed for use in the United States in the 1980s (such as the hepatitis B vaccine), the 1990s (such as the varicella vaccine), or later. The human papillomavirus (HPV) vaccine and the adults-only zoster (shingles) vaccine were licensed in 2006. Even if all an adult's shots are up to date, a yearly influenza vaccination may still be recommended. The fact is, if you haven't received a vaccination in the past few years, you probably need one!

As adults grow older, they start to lose some of their ability to fight off common infections. A bout of influenza that made you miss a few days of work in your 20s might lead to a hospital stay if you catch it in your 60s. Also, chances of developing a chronic illness or medical problem—such as diabetes or heart disease—increase as you get older. Some adult vaccinations can help protect you from infections that can be especially dangerous if you have other medical problems.

> ### Vaccinating Facts
>
> Thanks to a successful nationwide vaccination campaign, children are far more likely to receive their recommended vaccinations than adults. About 80 percent of children receive all their recommended childhood vaccines, and over 90 percent of children receive at least some of these vaccinations. Adult vaccination rates, on the other hand, are as low as about 25 percent against some diseases. As a result, adults account for about 95 percent of the cases of vaccine-preventable diseases in the United States, according to the CDC.

Vaccinations for Young Adults

Three vaccines are especially important for young adults (in their late teens and twenties): the Tdap (tetanus, diphtheria, and acellular pertussis) vaccine, the meningococcal vaccine, and the HPV (human papillomavirus) vaccine. Learn more specifics about each of these vaccines in Chapter 6.

Health Advisory

As with children, tell your doctor if you have ever had a life-threatening reaction to a vaccine dose or to a vaccine ingredient. You might not be able to receive some vaccinations. If you are somewhat or very ill with an acute illness on the day you are scheduled to receive a vaccination, tell your doctor. The vaccination might be postponed until you feel better.

People who did not receive the Tdap booster shot in adolescence should receive it as young adults (if they were never vaccinated against tetanus and diphtheria, they should get a three-dose primary vaccination against these diseases first). This vaccine provides protection against three sometimes-fatal types of bacterial infections. Before the vaccination, people should talk to their doctor if they have had seizures; a coma; epilepsy; problems with their nervous system; Guillain-Barré syndrome (GBS); or had a bad response to a previous dose of a vaccination against tetanus, diphtheria, and/or pertussis. The possible side effects from Tdap and Td vaccination—such as pain or swelling at the injection site, fever, headache, and nausea or digestive problems—are similar in both adults and children.

If a person did not receive a meningococcal vaccine when he or she was younger, it is important to receive one now. Meningococcal disease can lead to a rapidly developing, life-threatening bacterial infection in young adults, including bacterial meningitis (brain infection). Because it is spread by kissing, sharing food, coughing, and sneezing, people who live in close quarters (such as in dormitories or military barracks) are at increased risk for meningococcal disease. Young adults should receive the one-dose meningococcal conjugate vaccine (MCV4). Before the vaccination, adults should advise their doctor if they have had Guillain-Barré Syndrome (GBS) in the past. Very rarely, GBS has occurred after an MCV4 vaccination. Preteens, adolescents, and adults have similar possible side effects after the vaccination, such as pain at the injection site and fever.

Young women who did not receive their HPV vaccinations as preteens or adolescents should be vaccinated by age 26. The HPV vaccination can help prevent cervical cancer, genital warts, and other problems caused by four subtypes of sexually transmitted HPV viruses (the HPV vaccine will probably be recommended for young men as well in the near future). The vaccine is given in three doses over six months. The second dose should be given two months after the first dose, and the third dose should be given at least six months after the first dose.

A woman should not be vaccinated if she has a severe yeast allergy. Preteens, adolescents, and adults have similar possible side effects after the vaccination, such as pain, swelling, redness, or itching at the injection site or fever.

Brain Booster

Military recruits often live in close quarters, travel abroad, and might be exposed to biological weapons. For this reason, they might need certain travel vaccinations and vaccinations against pathogens such as anthrax, as well as the standard vaccinations currently recommended for young adults.

Young adults should also make sure that their vaccinations are up to date for these diseases as well:

◆ Hepatitis B

◆ Measles, mumps, and rubella (MMR)

◆ Polio

◆ Varicella (chickenpox)

◆ Hepatitis A

◆ Influenza (recommended yearly if living in a dormitory or other highly populated space)

◆ Pneumococcal disease (if certain health problems exist)

Vaccinations for All Adults

It's important for all adults to create or maintain immunity to a number of diseases, including tetanus, diphtheria, and pertussis (Td and Tdap vaccines); varicella (chickenpox); and measles, mumps, and rubella (MMR vaccine). Depending on age and health, adults might also need a yearly influenza vaccination. Adults age 60 and over should receive several additional vaccinations, discussed later in this chapter.

Health Advisory _____

Have you adopted a child internationally? Hepatitis B is a common infection in many parts of the world, including Asia and Africa. Your adopted child should be tested for hepatitis B so that he or she can receive optimal medical care. If your child does have a hepatitis B infection, you and your family members (and anyone else who has close contact with your child) should get a hepatitis B vaccination as well.

Td/Tdap Vaccination in Adults

All adults need to maintain their immunity to tetanus, diphtheria, and pertussis by receiving booster shots every 10 years. For those who have only been vaccinated with Td (the tetanus and diphtheria vaccine) in the past, and never received a dose of Tdap (the tetanus, diphtheria, and acellular pertussis vaccine), they should receive one Tdap dose in place of their next Td booster to establish immunity to pertussis. They should then receive a booster dose of Td every 10 years.

If an adult has never received a Td or Tdap vaccination, he or she should receive a three-dose vaccination as an adult. One of the doses can be Td or Tdap, and the other two doses should be Td. The second dose should be received at least 4 weeks after the first dose, and the third dose should be received 6 to 12 months after the second dose. After that, an adult needs a booster dose of Td every 10 years to maintain immunity. If he or she never received a dose of Tdap, one of the booster doses should be Tdap instead of Td.

It is especially important for adults to be vaccinated against tetanus and pertussis. Tetanus infections are more often fatal in older people than in younger people. Pertussis, which can cause a chronic cough in adults, can be fatal to babies who are not yet vaccinated against it. Adults who live with or care for an infant could pass pertussis on to the infant.

Before vaccination, adults should consult a doctor if they have had seizures, a coma, epilepsy, problems with their nervous system, or Guillain-Barré syndrome (GBS), or if they had a bad response to a previous dose of a vaccination against tetanus, diphtheria, and/or pertussis. The possible side effects from Tdap and Td vaccination, such as pain or swelling at the injection site, fever, headache, and nausea, are similar in both adults and children.

The Return of Chickenpox

In adults, chickenpox infections can cause severe complications, such as pneumonia. If you catch chickenpox as a child or an adult, the varicella (chickenpox) virus stays in your body after infection and can return years later and cause a painful rash called shingles. Adults who never had chickenpox or shingles, and who were never vaccinated against chickenpox, should get vaccinated as an adult. Varicella vaccination is also important for adults who live or work with someone who has a weakened immune system.

The two doses of the varicella vaccination should be separated by at least four weeks. Children and adults have similar potential side effects after the vaccination, including swelling at the injection site, fever, and rash. Before receiving the vaccine, adults should consult their doctor if an illness or drug treatment is affecting their immune system, if they have cancer or are being treated for cancer, or if they have received blood products recently. Adults should not get vaccinated if they have a severe allergy to gelatin or neomycin (an antibiotic).

Brain Booster

Adults born before 1980 (before the varicella vaccine became available) probably caught chickenpox in childhood and might not need to get a chickenpox vaccination. If you were born before 1980, talk to your doctor about whether you need the vaccination.

Measles, Mumps, and Rubella (MMR)

Adults who had measles, mumps, and rubella in the past do not need to get the MMR vaccine (a blood test will show if you are immune to these diseases). If adults are not immune to all three diseases, however, they need to be vaccinated against them. It's important to have immunity to measles, mumps, and rubella because measles is extremely contagious, both measles and mumps can be very dangerous, and rubella can harm a pregnant woman's baby.

Adults born on or after 1957 who did not receive the MMR vaccination or catch these diseases in childhood should be vaccinated now. Those born before 1957 were probably exposed to measles and mumps and have immunity to these diseases, but not to rubella. For these people, a doctor might give one MMR dose to ensure immunity to all three diseases. People born on or after 1957 who were only partially vaccinated against these diseases might receive one dose of MMR. If a blood test shows that a woman who might have children does not have immunity to rubella, she should receive one MMR dose as well.

In some cases, adults might need two MMR doses if they do not have adequate immunity to these diseases. With two doses, the second dose should be given at least four weeks after the first one.

The CDC especially recommends a two-dose MMR vaccination for healthy adults if:

- They received a killed (inactivated) version of the measles vaccine, or an unknown type of measles vaccine, before 1968, because the inactivated measles vaccine did not create immunity to measles.

- There is an outbreak of measles or mumps in their area.

- They are not immune to these diseases and are a student in a school.

- They are not immune to these diseases and work in health care.

- They are not immune to these diseases and plan to travel abroad or go on a cruise. (Learn more about travel vaccinations in Chapter 10.)

- They are not immune to these diseases and might become pregnant.

Children, adolescents, and adults have similar possible side effects after the vaccination, such as fever, rash, joint pain and stiffness, and (rarely) seizures or bleeding problems. Teens and adult women are more likely to feel temporary joint pain or stiffness.

If adults have had a severe reaction to gelatin or to neomycin, they should not get an MMR vaccination. An adult should consult a doctor if an illness or drug treatment is affecting his or her immune system, if he or she has cancer or is being treated for cancer, or if he or she has had problems with their blood or received blood products.

The Flu Shot

Because influenza can be especially harmful to older adults, all adults age 50 and over should receive one flu shot each year. Even if one is under 50 years old, it's a good idea to get a flu shot when living with or caring for a child under 5 years old, a person 50 or older, or someone with a chronic illness, or if you live in a nursing home or other special care facility. Many adults under 50 choose to get a flu shot simply to avoid catching influenza each year. It is best to get the vaccination in October or November, before flu season begins each year.

As we talked about in Chapters 4 and 6, there are two types of influenza vaccines: inactivated and live. The inactivated (injected) flu shot is best for adults ages 50 or older who have chronic health problems, who spend time with individuals who have weakened immune systems, or who live in nursing homes and special care facilities. The live (nasal spray) vaccine is only approved for healthy children and adults under 50 years old. To get the live vaccine, adults must not have a severe nasal problem or live with or care for someone with a weakened immune system.

Before vaccination, adults should consult their doctors if they are severely allergic to eggs, monosodium glutamate (MSG, a food additive), arginine (an amino acid sometimes used to treat certain medical conditions), gentamicin (an antibiotic), or gelatin, or if they have had Guillain-Barré syndrome (GBS). These individuals might not be able to get the influenza vaccination. The possible side effects from the flu shot are swelling at the injection site, fever, and achiness; the possible side effects from the live nasal spray include temporary flulike symptoms such as a runny nose, cough, chills, or a sore throat.

Shots for Seniors

As you age, your body's immune system becomes less effective. You become more vulnerable to disease, making vaccination even more important. People ages 65 and older should continue to receive inactivated influenza injections each year, and Td booster shots every 10 years. They should make sure they have immunity to chickenpox, measles, mumps, and rubella as well. Older adults should ask their health-care providers whether they need to be vaccinated against meningococcal disease, hepatitis A, and hepatitis B based on their health, lifestyle, occupation, and other factors.

Two other vaccines are recommended specifically for older adults: a zoster vaccine to prevent shingles and a PPV to prevent pneumonia, blood infection, and other problems. Shingles and pneumococcal infections can be very dangerous for older adults; unfortunately, many older adults don't receive these important vaccinations.

Varicella Zoster (Shingles)

The varicella virus, also called the varicella zoster virus or the herpes zoster virus, that causes chickenpox can sometimes cause a very painful skin rash called *shingles* that develops many years after a chickenpox infection. People can get shingles at any age, but it is most common in older adults and in people with weakened immune systems.

def•i•ni•tion

> The varicella virus that causes chickenpox can also cause an illness called **shingles,** usually in older adults. Shingles can cause a rash and severe nerve pain.

The shingles rash often appears on the trunk of the body or the face. Pain from the rash can be so severe that it is difficult for the adult to function. The rash usually goes away within a month, but for about 20 percent of adults who get shingles, the pain persists for weeks or months. For some very ill people, shingles can also cause pneumonia, among other health problems.

Chances of getting shingles increase as people get older. Adults can only get shingles if they had chickenpox or a chickenpox vaccine when they were younger. Shingles caused by the chickenpox vaccine are usually much milder than shingles caused by a chickenpox infection. If someone does develop shingles, he or she might infect others with chickenpox.

The one-dose shingles vaccine (a live, attenuated vaccine) was licensed in 2006 for adults age 60 or older. It is similar to the varicella (chickenpox) vaccine, but it contains a much greater amount of the weakened virus. Shingles vaccination can cause a headache or pain or itching at the injection site.

Vaccinating Facts

Vaccines you receive as an adult tend to be less effective than vaccines you receive as a child. For example, the shingles vaccine is about 65 percent effective at preventing shingles in adults ages 60 to 69 according to the CDC, although it can make a shingles infection less severe if it does occur. It is less effective in adults age 70 and older. Most childhood vaccines, by contrast, are at least 80 percent effective at preventing disease.

People with a severe allergy to gelatin or neomycin should not receive the shingles vaccine. Adults should consult a doctor if they have an illness that weakens their immune system, are taking drugs that weaken the immune system, have cancer or untreated tuberculosis, are being treated for cancer, or have received blood products.

Pneumococcal Polysaccharide Vaccine (PPV)

Pneumococcal bacteria can cause lung, blood, and brain infections. Most cases of pneumonia are caused by pneumococcal bacteria. Unfortunately, many of the bacteria have become resistant to antibiotics, making these infections difficult to treat.

Pneumococcal infections are more likely to be fatal in older adults than in younger adults. Adults 65 or older should get one PPV dose, unless they have received a dose of the vaccine within the past five years. If they have certain medical conditions, they might need a second dose as well.

Adults receive a PPV, an inactivated vaccine which is structured differently than the children's pneumococcal conjugate vaccine (PCV). The PPV protects adults from 23 types of bacteria that cause almost 90 percent of pneumococcal infections in adults. It was licensed in the United States in 1983.

After the vaccination, adults may feel side effects such as swelling or pain at the injection site or a fever for a few days.

Adults with Health Problems

Adults might need some extra vaccinations if they have a chronic illness or medical condition. Often vaccinations are less effective when a chronic illness is present, but they can still provide some protection.

Adults who have a disease or are receiving medical treatments that weaken their immune system might need to avoid live vaccines. Live vaccines given to adults include the varicella (chickenpox) vaccine, the zoster (shingles) vaccine, the MMR vaccine, and the live influenza vaccine.

People with a chronic illness or medical condition should consult a doctor as to whether they might need these additional vaccinations as well:

- PPV, if you are under 65 years old

- Hepatitis A (also available for adults as a combination vaccine with hepatitis B)

- Hepatitis B

- Influenza vaccine

- Meningococcal conjugate vaccine (MCV4, generally recommended for adults up to age 55) or meningococcal polysaccharide vaccine (MPSV4, used for adults over 55)

- Hib (*Haemophilus influenzae* type b), if you have your spleen removed or have certain other medical problems

Vaccinations and Pregnancy

Women planning to become pregnant should ask their doctor whether their vaccinations are up to date. If any vaccinations are needed, it's best to get them at least three months before becoming pregnant. If necessary, however, women can get some other vaccinations just one month before becoming pregnant.

It is especially important for a woman to find out whether she needs a vaccination against rubella (an MMR vaccination) or varicella (chickenpox). Both of these viruses can cause birth defects if caught while pregnant. Because the MMR and varicella vaccines are live vaccines, women should not receive them while pregnant (in most cases).

Before becoming pregnant, a doctor will give a woman a blood test that checks her immunity to rubella and hepatitis B. She will receive vaccinations against these diseases if needed.

If a woman finds out she is not immune to rubella or varicella after becoming pregnant, she should avoid contact with anyone who has these illnesses. After the baby is born, the mother will receive an MMR or varicella vaccination as needed. If the mother has hepatitis B, the baby will receive a standard hepatitis B vaccination just after birth, as well as a dose of hepatitis B immune globulin (a blood product that contains antibodies to hepatitis B) to help prevent infection.

Two vaccines are sometimes recommended for pregnant women: the inactivated influenza vaccine and a tetanus booster (usually the Td vaccine). If possible, it's best to avoid all other vaccines while pregnant.

Pregnant women should get an influenza vaccination if they will be pregnant during the winter months, because influenza can be especially severe in pregnant women. The inactivated influenza vaccination is safe for pregnant women and can protect her and the baby from influenza complications.

If a pregnant woman's Td or Tdap vaccination is out of date, or if she was never vaccinated against tetanus, diphtheria, or pertussis, she should get a booster dose of Td or Tdap or begin a series of primary doses. She can have this vaccination during pregnancy if necessary because it's very important for her to pass on antibodies to these diseases to her newborn. The Td dose is usually recommended for pregnant women, but the Tdap might be necessary if the mother is at risk for catching pertussis. It's best to get a Td or Tdap vaccination or start the series of doses after the first trimester of pregnancy.

There is limited data available about the effect of most vaccines on pregnancy. A doctor might recommend that a pregnant woman get an inactivated vaccine, though, if a woman is at special risk for a certain disease or if there is an outbreak of a disease in the area. Inactivated vaccines include the hepatitis A vaccine; the hepatitis B vaccine; the HPV vaccine (although it's best to avoid this vaccine while pregnant); the MCV4 or MPSV4; the PPV; the inactivated polio vaccine (IPV); and the Td or Tdap vaccine.

The rabies vaccine might be medically necessary for women who had contact with an animal with rabies before or after becoming pregnant. Learn more about this inactivated vaccine in Chapters 9 and 10. Also, if a pregnant woman plans to leave the country, there are other vaccines to consider for travel, covered in Chapter 10.

Vaccinating Facts
The CDC and many vaccine manufacturers keep track of the effect of certain vaccines on pregnancy. If you receive a vaccination (aside from the inactivated influenza vaccination) while pregnant, or a month or sooner before you become pregnant, ask your doctor whether to report this information and other data about your pregnancy to the CDC or the vaccine manufacturer. This data will help researchers learn more about the risks and benefits of vaccines during pregnancy.

Pregnant women should avoid receiving live vaccines because, in theory, these vaccines could harm the developing fetus. They are not recommended for pregnant women simply because they usually have not been tested in pregnant women. But, women who have accidentally received live vaccines before they knew they were pregnant have had healthy babies.

Women who are breastfeeding can safely receive any inactivated or live vaccine, except for the smallpox vaccine. In general, both inactivated and live vaccines are considered safe for healthy nursing mothers and their infants.

Vaccinations for Health-Care Workers

Health-care workers need certain vaccinations to protect themselves from infection and to avoid spreading infectious diseases to patients.

Health-care workers and volunteers in health-care settings should receive an influenza vaccination yearly, regardless of their age. When working with people with very suppressed immune systems, adults should get the inactivated (killed) influenza vaccine rather than the live (LAIV) vaccine.

Like all adults, health-care workers should receive booster shots to protect against tetanus, diphtheria, and pertussis. One of the adult booster shots should be Tdap (tetanus, diphtheria, and acellular pertussis), and the rest of the shots can be Td (tetanus and diphtheria).

Health-care workers who do not have immunity to varicella (chicken-pox) should receive the two-dose varicella vaccination. Those ages 60 and over should receive the varicella zoster vaccine as well to prevent shingles. Health-care workers should also follow the adult recommendations for MMR vaccination to make sure they have immunity to measles, mumps, and rubella.

In most cases, health-care workers should be vaccinated against hepatitis B as well with the three-dose vaccine. The second dose should be given one month after the first dose, and the third dose should be given six months after the first dose.

Health Advisory

Any researchers who work with pathogens that cause vaccine-preventable disease in adults, or who work with animals infected with these pathogens, should be vaccinated against the disease. For example, if you work with the bacteria that cause meningococcal disease or the virus that causes smallpox, you should get vaccinated against these diseases.

Anyone who works with the *Neiserria meningititis* bacterium should receive the meningococcal vaccine as well. People 55 and younger should receive one dose of the MCV4 vaccine, and those over 55 should receive the MPSV4 vaccine.

Other Groups

Adults should tell their doctors what they do for work, their lifestyle, their ethnicity, and the health and age of the people around them. They might need to get some vaccinations to protect everyone in the situation from harm. The following chart lists the important vaccinations that some groups of people might need.

Vaccinations for Specific Groups

If You ...	You Should Be Current on These Vaccinations:
... work with children under 12 months old	Tdap, varicella (chickenpox), influenza (yearly)
... teach or care for children	Varicella, influenza (yearly)
... are developmentally disabled, or work with developmentally disabled people	Hepatitis B, influenza
... are a college student	Varicella, MMR, meningococcal, influenza
... are in the military	Varicella, meningococcal, influenza, and possibly smallpox, anthrax, and the travel vaccinations
... live with or care for someone 65 or older	Influenza (yearly)
... work with patients in health care	Tdap, varicella, MMR, influenza (yearly), hepatitis B
... smoke or have asthma	Pneumococcal polysaccharide (PPSV), influenza
... are an American Indian, an Alaska native, or 50 years old or older	Pneumococcal polysaccharide (PPSV), Hib
... work in public safety	Hepatitis B, influenza
... have a sexually transmitted disease or engage in risky sexual behavior	Hepatitis B
... are a man who has sex with other men	Hepatitis A

Vaccinations Important for Adults

Age Group	Vaccination
Young adults	Tdap: booster shot
	Meningococcal vaccine (MCV4), one dose
	HPV vaccine, three doses over 6 or more months
	Influenza, yearly when have certain health, living, or work circumstances
Mid-aged adults	Td booster every 10 years
	Varicella, two doses at least 4 weeks apart if not immune to chickenpox
	MMR: one to two doses, at least 4 weeks apart, if not immune to measles, mumps, and rubella
Older adults	Td, every 10 years
	Influenza, yearly for ages 50 and over
	Varicella zoster (shingles): one dose at age 60 or older
	Pneumococcal polysaccharide vaccine (PPV): one dose at age 65 or older

The Least You Need to Know

◆ Adults should get many of the childhood vaccines that have been licensed in recent years.

◆ Adults need regular influenza and tetanus vaccinations throughout their lives.

◆ Seniors should get a shingles vaccination and a PPV vaccination.

◆ Health-care workers might need extra vaccinations.

◆ If possible, pregnant women should avoid live vaccines.

Part 3

Episodic and Circumstantial Vaccinations

Some vaccinations aren't part of the standard vaccination schedule. People with certain injuries might need special protective vaccinations. People who work in health care or the military might need vaccinations to better respond to a bioterrorist threat. International travelers might need to get a recommended or required vaccine before they go abroad. This part describes special and important vaccines that are not part of the standard vaccination schedule. This part also explains vaccines that are being developed for future use, such as vaccines for malaria and cancer.

Chapter 8

Vaccinations for ill Children and Adults

In This Chapter

- How acutely and chronically ill people can be vaccinated
- Illnesses or allergies that might prevent getting a vaccination
- Extra vaccinations some ill children and adults might need

What happens if your immune system is already battling an illness or is weakened by a disease or medical treatment? And what if you are severely allergic to an ingredient in a vaccine?

In most cases, vaccines are safe to get even if you are ill. They can help protect ill people even when they are most vulnerable to disease. In fact, some vaccines are specifically recommended for people with chronic illnesses. But, keep in mind that in some cases, a vaccine can be harmful for an ill person. Whether a vaccine is harmful for you depends on your own health history, your risk for catching a disease, and how the vaccine is made.

Acutely ill Children

If you are a parent, you probably know that young children get sick quite often. Most young children catch at least four or five colds a year, for example, with symptoms such as a runny nose, a mild fever, and sneezing. Colds and influenza are illnesses that last a short time—a few days to a few weeks. These are examples of *acute* illnesses. Yet when a medical problem lasts a long time, or comes and goes on a regular basis, it is called a *chronic* illness. Diabetes and asthma are two common chronic illnesses in children.

def•i•ni•tion

> An **acute** illness lasts for a short time period and usually does not have long-term health effects. A **chronic** illness is ongoing or comes and goes and can damage your overall health.

A child may have a cold or other acute illness when visiting the doctor for one of the routine childhood vaccinations. If this happens, the doctor should be told the child is sick, and also whether the child is taking any medications. It's usually safe to go ahead with the vaccination if the child has a mild acute illness such as a cold, low fever, diarrhea, or ear infection. If the child has a more severe illness, it's likely best to wait until he or she recovers before administering a vaccination—the doctor will recommend the best course of action. If it's necessary to postpone the vaccination, the appointment should be rescheduled to make sure the child gets the vaccination.

Depending on the circumstances, the doctor might go ahead and vaccinate the child even if he or she has an acute illness. The child might need the vaccination now if he or she is not available for another appointment soon enough, or if there is an outbreak of a vaccine-preventable disease in the community. In most cases, getting the vaccination will not harm the child. If an acutely ill child develops a problem such as a high fever after the vaccination, however, it is difficult to determine whether it was caused by the illness or by the vaccination. That is why it's usually better (if not always possible) to postpone a vaccination until the child feels better.

Chronically ill Children

When a child has a chronic illness such as asthma or a blood disorder or is receiving long-term medical therapies, discuss the health issues with the child's doctor. The doctor will assess the child's medical history and risk of being exposed to a vaccine-preventable disease. In most cases, a doctor will recommend going ahead with the vaccination because, if a chronically ill child catches a vaccine-preventable disease such as chickenpox, the disease can be much worse for the child than for a healthy child. And, while a vaccination is sometimes less effective in a chronically ill child, it can still provide some protection against disease. Unless he or she has a weakened immune system, usually a chronically ill child can get vaccinations on the same schedule as a healthy child.

Health Advisory

Are vaccines safe for premature and low birth weight infants? The first dose of the hepatitis B vaccination, given at birth to full-term infants, is sometimes delayed one month for low birth weight infants. In most cases, however, premature and low birth weight infants can receive all their standard vaccinations on the same schedule as full-term infants. The vaccination schedule follows the infant's chronological age, not his or her corrected age (the age based on developmental level). For example, at the two-month pediatric visit, a premature infant will most likely receive the same vaccinations as a two-month-old full-term infant: the hepatitis B, rotavirus, DTaP, Hib, pneumococcal (PCV7), and polio (IPV) vaccines.

If a child has an illness that weakens his or her immune system (such as AIDS) or is taking long-term medications that weaken his or her immune system (such as steroids), the child might need to skip or delay vaccination with any live (attenuated) vaccines. These live vaccines include the measles, mumps, and rubella (MMR) vaccine; the varicella (chickenpox) vaccine; and the live influenza vaccine (recommended for children two years and older). If a child's immune system is very weak, a live vaccine could cause medical complications rather than preventing disease. A child's doctor might decide to delay or skip certain vaccinations if he or she has other medical issues, such as neurological problems, or is having long-term aspirin treatments.

> **Health Advisory**
>
> Like children, adolescents and adults can usually receive vaccinations even if they have a mild illness such as a cold. Moderately to seriously ill adolescents and adults—with an acute illness (such as a sinus infection) or a chronic illness (such as heart disease or diabetes)—and those taking long-term medications (such as steroids) should discuss their health history with their doctor before they receive a vaccination. Adults with immune system problems might need to avoid the live vaccines: MMR, varicella (chickenpox), LAIV (influenza), and varicella zoster (shingles).

High-Risk Groups

Children, adolescents, and adults with certain medical problems might receive special vaccinations in addition to the standard vaccinations to protect them from dangerous infections.

Pneumococcal disease is a special risk for chronically ill children, adolescents, and adults. This bacterial disease can cause lung, blood, or brain infections, and it has become resistant to many antibiotics, which is why it is important to prevent it through vaccinations.

> **Health Advisory**
>
> Even if you have all your recommended vaccinations, remember that your health and health-care needs might change over time. If you are diagnosed with a new health problem such as heart disease or kidney failure, ask your health-care provider whether you might need extra vaccinations to protect your health.

All children should receive a four-dose vaccination against pneumococcal disease by the time they are 15 months old. The pneumococcal conjugate vaccine (PCV7) is formulated to be effective in young children. People between ages 2 and 65 years old with certain health problems sometimes need one or two doses of a different type of pneumococcal vaccine, called the pneumococcal polysaccharide vaccine

(PPV23). If two PPV23 doses are needed, they are usually given three to five years apart. A child or adult may need a PPV23 vaccination if he or she has a chronic health problem (such as heart disease or diabetes), if he or she has a cochlear implant, if the individual has an illness that weakens the immune system, or if the individual is receiving medical treatments that weaken the immune system (such as radiation therapy). Pneumococcal disease is also a risk for people who smoke.

Chronically ill adults might need to extend their yearly influenza vaccinations (the inactivated vaccine only) because complications from influenza can be worse in ill people than in healthy people. The vaccine is currently recommended for all children up to age 18 and for all adults 50 years of age and older. But, if you have a chronic illness or medical condition and are between 18 and 50, you might need to receive a yearly influenza vaccination.

Health Advisory

Healthy people who live with or care for someone with a chronic illness should get a yearly influenza vaccination. Either the live (LAIV) or inactivated influenza vaccination is okay unless the chronically ill person has a severely weakened immune system (then you should not have the LAIV). Consult a doctor about the other vaccinations needed to protect everyone's health.

Some people might also need to get a hepatitis A vaccine. Hepatitis A, as discussed in Chapter 5, is a viral liver disease that can cause severe illness. The two-dose hepatitis A vaccination is recommended for all children between one and two years of age. Older children and adults with chronic liver disease or certain blood disorders should receive the hepatitis A vaccination if they do not already have immunity to the disease through a previous vaccination or infection.

Hepatitis B infections, which can be acute or chronic and lead to serious medical problems, are also a risk for people with liver or kidney problems or HIV infection. People with one of these illnesses who have not received hepatitis B vaccinations in the past might need the multidose vaccination now.

Bacterial meningitis, which can cause brain damage and other problems, is another high risk for certain chronically ill people, such as those with certain immune system problems. The standard one-dose meningococcal conjugate vaccine (MCV4, discussed in Chapter 6) is usually given at adolescence (11 to 12 years old), and a meningococcal polysaccharide vaccine (MPSV4) is sometimes used for adults over 55. But, a chronically ill child might receive an MCV4 vaccine at age two, and a chronically ill adult might receive one or more doses of the MCV4 or MPSV4 vaccine to help ensure protection.

In some cases, an older child or adult might need to be vaccinated against *Haemophilus influenzae* type b (Hib) with a three- or four-dose Hib vaccine. Hib infections, which can lead to bacterial meningitis and other problems, are a risk for people with HIV/AIDS and a risk for people undergoing medical procedures such as certain cancer treatments, bone marrow transplants, or spleen removal.

Allergies

Children, adolescents, and adults sometimes have environmental allergies such as hay fever or moderate (yet not life-threatening) food allergies. If adults or children have these allergies, they can likely still get all their recommended vaccinations.

Vaccinating Facts

Allergy shots, also called immunotherapy, are similar to vaccines because they train your immune system to become immune to the allergens that cause allergies. Allergy shots contain a small amount of an allergen, and the amount is gradually increased to help your body learn to tolerate an allergen. To be effective, allergy shots must be given every few weeks for several years. Allergy shots can reduce or prevent some types of allergies, but they can't be used to prevent food allergies.

A doctor should be told if any life-threatening allergies have occurred in the past. Some vaccines contain substances that could trigger these allergies. For example, the influenza vaccine is grown in chicken egg cells, and yeast cells are used to make the hepatitis B vaccine and the human papillomavirus (HPV) vaccine. Some vaccines contain antibiotics such as neomycin to prevent contamination. Gelatin is used to stabilize some vaccines, and vaccines might be stored or administered in containers made of latex.

If a child or adult has a severe allergy to any of these substances, talk to the doctor before receiving any vaccinations:

- Alum (a vaccine adjuvant)
- Baker's yeast (baker's yeast cells are used to make certain vaccines)
- Eggs (some vaccines are grown in egg cells)
- Gelatin (a vaccine stabilizer)
- Latex (some vaccines are stored or administered in latex containers)
- Rodent or neural proteins (used rarely in vaccines)
- 2-phenoxyethanol (a vaccine preservative)
- Neomycin (an antibiotic)
- Polymyxin B (an antibiotic)
- Streptomycin (an antibiotic)
- Thimerosal (a vaccine preservative)

Although it happens very rarely, when someone has a life-threatening reaction to a dose of a vaccine, they should not receive another dose of that vaccine. This reaction, called anaphylaxis, can occur minutes after receiving the vaccination. Anaphylaxis usually begins with severe itchiness of the face or eyes. Hives, swelling, low blood pressure, stomach pain, vomiting, breathing problems, and choking can occur a few minutes later. Anaphylaxis is a medical emergency and needs immediate medical attention. This is why it is so important to tell the doctor about all allergies prior to any vaccination.

Vaccination Guidelines for Ill Children and Adults

Vaccines to avoid for those with weakened immune systems:

- ◆ MMR vaccine

- ◆ Varicella (chickenpox) vaccine

- ◆ Live influenza vaccine (LAIV)

- ◆ Varicella zoster (shingles) vaccine (older adults only)

Vaccines potentially needed for those with certain medical problems:

- ◆ Pneumococcal vaccine (PPV or PPSV)

- ◆ Influenza vaccine

- ◆ Hepatitis A vaccine

- ◆ Hepatitis B vaccine

- ◆ Meningococcal vaccine (MCV4 or MPSV4)

- ◆ Hib vaccine

The Least You Need to Know

- ◆ You can usually get a vaccination even if you have an acute illness.

- ◆ If you have a chronic illness, you might need some extra vaccinations to protect your health.

- ◆ It is very important to know about any allergies prior to receiving vaccinations due to the substances used in making and storing many vaccines.

Chapter 9

Special Vaccinations for Injuries or Bioterrorism

In This Chapter

- ◆ When an unscheduled tetanus vaccination is necessary
- ◆ When a rabies vaccination is necessary
- ◆ The three types of anthrax exposure
- ◆ When a smallpox vaccination is necessary

Even if you have all the vaccinations needed for your age and health criteria, sudden injuries or accidental exposure to certain bacteria and viruses could still put you at risk. There are four vaccines that are particularly helpful in combating exposure due to injuries or bioterrorism—a recent phenomenon—and, in this chapter, we'll talk about each one of them.

Tetanus

As you already know from Chapter 4, you can't catch tetanus from another person; you get it from the environment. Spores of the tetanus bacteria are in the environment all around us—in the soil, animal droppings, and manure. If they enter the bloodstream through an injury, they can cause a dangerous infection.

While a person can get a tetanus infection from stepping on a dirty nail that punctures the skin, there are many other ways of being exposed to keep in mind. You can also develop tetanus from a severe burn, frostbite, an animal bite, a tattoo, a dental infection, surgery, or even pregnancy. Illegal drug users who inject heroin sometimes get tetanus from the substances used to make heroin.

Tetanus infections are serious because they can cause symptoms such as high blood pressure, fever, sweating, and severe muscle spasms such as lockjaw (spasms of the jaw muscles). Sometimes, these muscle spasms are strong enough to fracture a bone, and they can become life-threatening if they occur in the throat or in the muscles that help you breathe. As a result, about 30 percent of people in the United States who develop tetanus die from it.

Cleaning and covering any wounds—even small scrapes, scratches, and splinters—can decrease the chances of developing tetanus, but regular tetanus vaccinations are still needed to ensure protection. In some tetanus cases among unvaccinated people, the infected person does not know how they got tetanus.

The standard diphtheria, tetanus, and acellular pertussis (DTaP) vaccination series received in childhood will keep children protected, and adolescents and adults should have tetanus and diphtheria (Td) vaccinations every 10 years (one of which should be Tdap).

When You Might Need It

When a person is injured badly enough to seek medical help, the doctor will ask about the person's tetanus vaccination history. Tetanus incubates in the body for a few days or weeks before symptoms develop.

Vaccination after an injury, before the bacteria releases its toxins in your bloodstream, can prevent or diminish tetanus symptoms.

Health Advisory

Before receiving any vaccination, tell your doctor if you (or your child) have had a life-threatening reaction to a dose of a vaccine or to a vaccine ingredient, or if you are moderately or very ill with an acute illness. If you or your child need to receive a vaccine due to an injury or bioterrorism, your doctor will discuss the risks and benefits of this decision. In many cases, getting the vaccine, even if you are pregnant or have a chronic illness, is the safest choice.

If the person's tetanus vaccinations are up to date and he or she has received a booster within the past five years, then there is protection after an injury. If the vaccinations are not up to date and no tetanus shot has been received in the past five years, the doctor will give the person one (DTaP, Td, or Tdap, depending on the age and vaccination history). Although tetanus vaccinations provide immunity for 10 years for most people, immunity wears off in less than 10 years for some. Therefore, a tetanus shot after the injury will provide protection in case the immunity to tetanus did not last 10 years.

What if someone is injured and has never been vaccinated against tetanus, or hasn't completed the recommended vaccinations? In these cases, a person would receive a tetanus shot (Td or Tdap) and a dose of tetanus immune globulin—a blood product that contains tetanus antibodies and provides temporary immunity. These actions might diminish or prevent the effects of a tetanus infection.

Health Advisory

Tetanus is different than other diseases because, if you catch and recover from tetanus, you do *not* develop any immunity to it. You can still get tetanus in the future, even if you've had it in the past. For that reason, keep getting your booster shots, which will ensure your immunity to tetanus.

Side Effects and Problems

When an adult needs a tetanus, diphtheria, and acellular pertussis (Tdap) or Td vaccination after an injury, the doctor needs to know if there is a history of severe latex allergy, epilepsy or other seizures, nervous system problems or coma, or a history of Guillain-Barré Syndrome (GBS). A Td or Tdap vaccination can cause pain or swelling at the injection site, headache, fatigue, nausea, and other problems.

In rare cases, the arm where the shot has been administered can swell and become very painful within a few hours of the shot. This is more common in adults who have had a number of booster shots containing tetanus and diphtheria vaccines.

If a child needs a DTaP vaccination after an injury (given only to children under seven years old), the doctor needs to know of any nervous system or brain problems (such as confusion, headaches, vision changes, or dizziness), seizures, excessive crying, or high fever after any previous DTaP doses. The child may need to receive a different type of tetanus vaccination.

Rabies

Rabies is a virus that animals can give to humans. It is transmitted through the animal's saliva, usually by a bite. Sometimes an individual can catch rabies if an animal with rabies licks his or her nose or mouth, or licks an individual's open wound. The rabies virus can incubate in the body for several months or longer before symptoms begin. If a person is exposed to rabies and receives a vaccination during this incubation period, they will be protected from rabies. Once symptoms begin, however, the vaccination won't work. The symptoms of rabies include seizures and hallucinations, and rabies is fatal to humans.

Rabies is a public health issue because the number and type of animals with rabies varies by region. Local health authorities track rabies cases in their area so they can advise doctors about which animals are most likely to have it. An area with high rates of pet vaccinations against rabies, for example, likely makes it uncommon among domestic cats and dogs.

Rabies is most common among certain wild animals such as bats, raccoons (who might give rabies to unvaccinated cats), skunks, and foxes. Be careful if a bat gets in your house, because sometimes you might not be aware of a bat bite, or one could bite you in your sleep. Some exotic pets can also have rabies, even if a veterinarian has vaccinated them against rabies.

When You Might Need It

A person needs a rabies vaccination when he or she is bitten or licked by an animal that might have rabies. The wound should be thoroughly washed out to decrease the chances that some of the rabies virus, if the animal has it, could enter the blood. Then, a doctor or the public health department should be contacted right away to find out if there could be a risk for rabies. Rabies is rarely transmitted by licking, but if an animal is thought to be *rabid* and it licked the face or an open wound, consult a doctor right away.

> **def•i•ni•tion**
> A **rabid** animal is one that is infected with the rabies virus.

How can you tell if an animal is rabid? If an animal attacks without warning or is behaving oddly or looks ill, it might have rabies. If an animal is wounded and you don't know how it was wounded, it might have rabies as well because it was bitten or in contact with another animal with rabies.

If an animal is suspected of having rabies, it will be either euthanized and then examined for the disease or captured and observed for 10 days. If health authorities find that the animal does or probably has rabies and you were bitten or licked by the animal, you will need to get a rabies vaccination.

> **Brain Booster**
> People who regularly work with or are exposed to animals, such as veterinarians and animal researchers, often get a prophylactic (preventative) rabies vaccination. This type of vaccination is given before exposure to rabies.

The rabies vaccine is an inactivated vaccine. The current rabies vaccines were licensed in the United States in the 1980s and 1990s. The vaccine is given in five doses. The first injection is given right away, followed by doses 3, 7, 14, and 28 days later. If a person has never been vaccinated, he or she will also get a shot of rabies immune globulin to provide short-term protection from rabies. If a person has received a rabies vaccination in the past, he or she needs only two doses (one right after the incident, and one three days later) and no rabies immune globulin. The CDC might change this recommendation to a four-dose series in the near future (skipping the last dose). Researchers have found that four doses of the rabies vaccine are as effective as five doses.

Side Effects and Problems

A doctor needs to know if someone's immune system is weakened by disease such as HIV/AIDS or cancer, drug treatments, or cancer treatments, or if someone is taking antimalarial drugs. The rabies vaccine might be less effective in these cases.

After the vaccination, a person might feel sore at the injection site or have a headache, nausea, hives, or joint pain. Very rarely, a person develops GBS or other nervous system problems after a rabies vaccination.

Anthrax

Anthrax is a bacterial disease that can be transmitted from animals to people. Anthrax outbreaks can occur in livestock such as cattle, goats, sheep, camels, and other animals. These outbreaks are rare in the United States, where livestock are vaccinated against anthrax, but they do occur in other parts of the world.

People can catch anthrax if an infected animal product touches a cut on their skin—this is called cutaneous anthrax. People can also catch anthrax by eating undercooked infected meat, called gastrointestinal anthrax, or by inhaling anthrax spores, called inhalation anthrax. Any form of anthrax can be fatal if the blood or brain become infected, especially inhalation anthrax.

Cutaneous anthrax is the most common form of anthrax. It can be spread by contact with infected wool, hair, or animal hides. Its symptom is a sore that turns into a blister with a black center. Antibiotics can usually successfully treat cutaneous anthrax.

Gastrointestinal anthrax causes nausea, fever, and stomach pain, among other symptoms. Inhalation anthrax causes influenza-like symptoms and fever at first, but it can lead to shock, brain inflammation, and breathing problems. Antibiotics can sometimes help a patient recover from gastrointestinal or inhalation anthrax.

In 2001, inhalation anthrax was used as a biological weapon against 22 people in the United States. They inhaled anthrax spores and some died of the disease. Some believe anthrax could be used as a biological weapon again in the future.

An anthrax vaccine was licensed in the United States in 1970. It can prevent anthrax infection if it is given either before exposure to anthrax or before symptoms appear. The incubation period for anthrax is about one day to one week or more. The anthrax vaccine cannot cause anthrax.

When You Might Need It

The anthrax vaccine is used to protect people who might be exposed to anthrax through their occupation, such as researchers and some people in the military. It is only approved for adults 18 years old and older. You can learn more about the use of the anthrax vaccine in the United States military on the Department of Defense's Anthrax Vaccination Immunization Program website at www.anthrax.osd.mil.

Vaccinating Facts

The Centers for Disease Control and Prevention (CDC) maintains a Strategic National Stockpile of medical supplies, including antibiotics, antiviral medications, and vaccines, for use in a wide-scale emergency such as an earthquake or a terrorist attack. There is enough medicine in the Stragetic National Stockpile to meet the needs of several cities at the same time. If local authorities request the supplies, they can arrive within 12 hours of an emergency.

The anthrax vaccination involves five doses. The first two injections are given four weeks apart. The last three injections are given 6, 12, and 18 months after the first dose. After being vaccinated, a person needs to get a yearly booster dose to maintain immunity. If a large population were exposed to anthrax, they would probably be supplied with antibiotics to prevent infection, rather than vaccinated.

Side Effects and Problems

Soreness or a lump at the injection site is a common side effect from the vaccine. Sometimes, part of the arm where the injection was given also reddens. A person might experience muscle aches, headache, nausea, or other influenza-like symptoms after vaccination.

Brain Booster

Some soldiers who fought in the 1991 Persian Gulf War developed an illness called Gulf War Syndrome. It includes a range of symptoms, including fatigue, headaches, skin problems, and neurological problems. Some soldiers believed that the anthrax vaccine given to them during that war caused these symptoms, although this link has never been proven. The syndrome may have been caused by the soldiers' exposure to chemical weapons, burning oil, or other toxic substances used during the war.

New, recombinant versions of the anthrax vaccine are under development now (a technique described in Chapter 11). These new vaccines would require fewer doses and have fewer side effects than the current vaccine.

The anthrax vaccine is not known to cause illness in the men and women who have received the vaccine. If someone has had cutaneous anthrax, he or she should not receive the anthrax vaccine. Also, pregnant women should not receive the anthrax vaccine unless absolutely necessary.

Smallpox

As you know from Chapter 1, smallpox vaccinations, which used to be routinely recommended, are no longer needed. A global vaccination campaign eradicated smallpox worldwide by 1980.

The United States and Russia still keep some of the variola virus that causes smallpox in guarded laboratories. Several other countries are believed to have a supply of smallpox viruses as well. Because smallpox vaccinations are no longer routine, however, the population of the United States (among other countries) could be vulnerable to a biological attack of smallpox.

To prevent this, the U.S. government has created a stockpile of smallpox vaccines to vaccinate people in case they are deliberately exposed to smallpox. Researchers and teams of health-care and public health workers throughout the country are already vaccinated against smallpox so they can coordinate and provide vaccinations as needed if there were a biological attack.

When You Might Need It

Some members of the military, health-care workers, public health workers, and smallpox researchers already receive smallpox vaccinations. The one-dose vaccine is made from a live, attenuated virus that can create immunity to smallpox. There have been many versions of the smallpox vaccine in the past, but the current vaccine was licensed in 2007.

During vaccination, a person is quickly pricked several times with small needles. As the immune system reacts to the vaccine, the area where the vaccine was received blisters and scabs over. Until the scab falls off, special steps are needed to prevent the spread of the virus to others. The smallpox vaccination provides protection for 3 to 10 years, depending on the level of exposure to smallpox and related viruses.

In theory, some people should not receive this vaccination. People must be 18 years old or older to get the smallpox vaccination. In the case of individuals with heart problems, skin problems such as eczema or bad acne (or living with someone who has skin problems), or a weakened immune system from a disease or a medical treatment (or living with someone with a weakened immune system), the smallpox vaccination should not be given. Women who are pregnant (or individuals living with someone who is pregnant) or breastfeeding, or people who have severe allergies to latex or to the antibiotics polymyxin B, streptomycin, chlortetracycline, or neomycin should not get the vaccination. People might not be able to get the vaccinations if they have high blood pressure, high cholesterol, diabetes, relatives with certain heart conditions; take certain steroids; or smoke cigarettes.

If there were a smallpox outbreak, however, people might need to get the smallpox vaccine despite any risk factors they might have. In this case, the benefits of vaccination would probably outweigh the risks of catching smallpox, and public health officials would decide whether they needed to be vaccinated. If the vaccination is received within four days of being exposed to smallpox, it can often still protect a person from infection. If the vaccination is received four to seven days after exposure, it can diminish the effect of any smallpox infection.

Side Effects and Problems

Smallpox vaccination can cause a range of side effects, including fever, blisters, pain at the vaccination site, swollen lymph nodes, and a mild rash, usually within a day to two weeks of the vaccination. More severe but rare complications can include a severe rash, an inflamed heart, brain swelling, and other problems. Sometimes the vaccine can cause a mild, smallpox-like disease.

Vaccinations Used Against Injuries and Bioterrorism

Vaccine	Prevents	Dosage
DTaP, Td, or Tdap	Tetanus	One dose if last vaccination was more than 5 years ago; one dose plus a dose of tetanus immune globulin if never vaccinated
Rabies	Rabies	Five doses: one immediately and one 3, 7, 14, and 28 days after the injury, plus one dose of rabies immune globulin; if previously vaccinated, two doses are needed, one immediately and one three days after the injury (note that these recommendations might change to four doses)

Vaccine	Prevents	Dosage
Anthrax	Anthrax	Five doses: two doses 4 weeks apart, and doses 6, 12, and 18 months after; a yearly booster dose maintains immunity
Smallpox	Smallpox	One dose

The Least You Need to Know

◆ Many common injuries can lead to tetanus infections and require a tetanus booster shot.

◆ The risk of getting rabies and needing a rabies vaccination varies by region and type of animal.

◆ If you are exposed to anthrax, quick antibiotic treatment or vaccination can help prevent illness.

◆ The federal government has teams trained and ready to vaccinate the public if there is a biological attack using smallpox.

10

Vaccinations for Travelers

In This Chapter

- ◆ Resources and tips for planning a healthy trip
- ◆ Vaccinations needed for travel
- ◆ Protection from infectious diseases while you travel
- ◆ Diseases that are common in certain areas of the world

Routine vaccinations don't just protect you from diseases at home; they also protect you from getting ill when you travel to other countries because many vaccine-preventable diseases that are uncommon in the United States are common in other parts of the world. Before traveling, you also might need to get additional special vaccinations to protect you from other diseases, such as typhoid fever. It's best to plan ahead in getting any necessary vaccinations for travel. But, even if you have limited time before you go, your doctor can help you protect your health during your travels.

Before You Leave

When planning to travel to other countries, it's especially important to ensure you have received all your standard recommended vaccinations before you depart. Although you may never be exposed to a disease such as diphtheria or polio in the United States, outbreaks of these vaccine-preventable diseases still occur in other parts of the world. So, if you haven't updated your vaccinations lately, this is the time to do it. Depending on where and when you travel, you also might need some additional vaccinations that are not part of the standard U.S. vaccination schedule, such as vaccines that protect against yellow fever and typhoid fever.

Plan to see your doctor at least four to six weeks before traveling (several months before you leave is best). If you need vaccinations, you will have time to get all the required doses and your immune system will also have time to develop immunity to diseases for which you received vaccinations. If you're traveling to an area where malaria is common, you might need to start taking antimalarial drugs before you leave.

But what if you are leaving in less than a month? Talk to your doctor, because you might be able to receive some doses of a recommended vaccine and get some level of immunity to a disease. Your doctor also might decide to give you immune globulin for temporary protection from a disease, or to follow an accelerated schedule to give you all the doses you need of a vaccine before you leave. If you don't have time to follow the standard schedule, receiving all the doses of an important vaccination through an accelerated schedule might provide better protection than receiving a partial vaccination.

If you're planning international travel with children, they will also need updated vaccinations. Because so many vaccinations are given in childhood, however, your child might not yet have received all the doses of the vaccines he or she needs to be fully protected. Talk to your child's doctor about your international travel plans and the risks of vaccine-preventable diseases in the areas you plan to visit. Before you leave, your child might need to get some vaccinations—such as the measles, mumps, and rubella (MMR) vaccinations—on an accelerated schedule to ensure immunity to some diseases.

Brain Booster _____

Find out what travel coverage your health insurance offers before you go abroad. If you have a chronic condition, for example, your insurance might not cover illnesses related to your condition that happen when you travel. Generally, Medicare does not provide travel coverage. You may need to purchase extra medical coverage if you are planning international travel. Consider medical evacuation insurance as well, in case you need to be transported while ill. If you do need medical care while you travel, you will probably need to pay for the cost of care up front, and receive reimbursement from your insurer later. Also, be sure to bring a claim form and your medical insurance card with you when you travel abroad.

If your child is a newborn, you might need to postpone your trip, because no vaccine series except hepatitis B can be started before your child is six weeks old. Very young children may not be able to receive the vaccines recommended for travel—such as the yellow fever vaccine—because many travel vaccines are not recommended for children under one year old.

Finding CDC Recommendations

The Centers for Disease Control and Prevention (CDC) has a wealth of information for people planning to travel abroad, and it's all available online. Visit the Travelers' Health Destinations page on their website, wwwn.cdc.gov/travel/destinations/list.aspx, as you plan your trip. Here you will find travel notices and warnings about current disease outbreaks, information about the vaccines you might need to get before you go, and tips about traveling to specific countries or regions. The Travelers' Health page, wwwn.cdc.gov/travel/, provides general health and safety information for travelers. You can also call the CDC for information on countries you plan to visit: 1-877-FYI-TRIP or 1-877-394-8747.

The CDC has three types of vaccination recommendations:

1. **Routine vaccinations:** The standard vaccinations you should have as part of your regular health care, such as the MMR vaccination.

2. **Recommended vaccinations:** Optional vaccinations depending on your travel plans, health, age, vaccination history, and other factors. It is wise to learn about and get the CDC's recommended vaccinations, such as the typhoid fever vaccination, for a country or area you plan to visit.

3. **Required vaccinations:** Vaccinations that are not optional when traveling to certain countries or regions. Some countries require documents that prove you have certain vaccinations before you can enter the country. For example, you must have proof of a yellow fever vaccination to visit parts of Africa and South America. Saudi Arabia requires proof of meningococcal disease vaccination if you visit at certain times of the year.

To receive travel vaccinations, get vaccination documents, and make other health-related preparations for your trip, you may need to visit a health-care provider who specializes in travel medicine. This specialized care is especially helpful if you plan to visit several countries or areas, have a chronic health condition, or are pregnant. You can find a provider at a private travel medicine clinic or, in many states, at your local health department. To learn more about travel health-care providers, visit:

◆ The CDC's travel clinic page at wwwn.cdc.gov/travel/content/travel-clinics.aspx (or call 1-800-CDC-INFO)

◆ The International Society of Travel Medicine at www.istm.org (or call 770-736-7060)

◆ The American Society of Tropical Medicine and Hygiene at www.astmh.org (or call 847-480-9592)

The risks of encountering infectious diseases abroad are constantly changing. Some diseases are seasonal, with risks of infection varying depending on the time of year. Some diseases, such as *cholera*, can be eliminated or controlled with improved sanitation and healthy travel habits. Some diseases migrate with people; for example, meningococcal disease often breaks out during the annual Hajj, or pilgrimage to Mecca, in Saudi Arabia (the dates of the Hajj, based on the lunar Islamic calendar, vary each year). Other circumstances such as war, natural disasters, and other problems can also contribute to disease outbreaks.

Because the health risks of traveling abroad can change so often,
it's important to get updated
health information before you
travel abroad. The CDC provides
e-mail updates to keep up with
the latest health news; sign up
at www.cdc.gov/emailupdates/.
The U.S. Department of State
also offers country-specific travel
information (including health
information) online at http://
travel.state.gov.

def•i•ni•tion

Cholera is a bacterial disease that can cause severe
diarrhea, vomiting, and dehydration, and it can be fatal.
It is spread through contaminated food and drinks, and
is common in parts of Africa.
Currently, there is no vaccine
for cholera available in the
United States.

Tips for Healthy Travel

Infectious diseases can be spread in many ways. When you travel, you
can be exposed to an infectious disease through the food you eat; the
water you drink or swim in; bites from insects, such as mosquitoes;
contact with animals or animal droppings; sexual activity; contact with
body fluids; contact with soil containing certain bacterial spores; or by
breathing air near someone who has an infectious disease.

Even if you have all your routine, recommended, and required vaccinations when you travel, you still might develop a health problem. There
is no vaccine or medicine available to prevent many common infectious diseases such as the bacteria that cause travelers' diarrhea and the
viruses that cause gastroenteritis (vomiting and diarrhea), for example,
and injuries and accidents can happen at any time.

Brain Booster

Are you planning to go on a cruise? The CDC's Vessel Sanitation
Program (VSP) lists the sanitation scores and healthy travel tips for
cruise ships. A higher score indicates a cleaner ship. Better sanitation decreases your chance of catching an infectious disease on
board. Visit the VSP at www.cdc.gov/nceh/vsp/ and search the direc-
tory by the name of the cruise ship or by the cruise line.

Luckily, you can take many steps to stay healthy when you travel. Along with vaccinations, these commonsense tips can protect your health:

♦ Pack all the medicines you take regularly and might need on the trip. If possible, keep them in their original containers.

♦ Bring a letter from your health-care provider describing any medical condition that you have. The letter should list the generic names of any medications you take for it.

♦ Bring copies of your medicine and eyewear prescriptions, in case you need to fill them when you travel.

♦ Bring family members' immunization records for those traveling with you.

♦ Bring a copy of family members' medical histories.

♦ Keep children's toys and pacifiers clean.

♦ Be careful and mindful when on buses, motorcycles, bicycles, and other transportation. Use seatbelts and helmets as needed. Avoid overloaded transportation, and ask for help if you need to travel at night.

♦ Bring your child's car seat from home if you won't be able to rent a safe one.

♦ Wash your hands and your children's hands often.

♦ Take any malaria medicine as directed, if you will be traveling in an area where malaria is common.

Health Advisory

Malaria is caused by a parasite spread by mosquitoes. Its flulike symptoms include fever, muscle aches, and fatigue. Malaria can cause jaundice and serious problems, such as seizures, and it can be fatal. The disease is very common in the Southern Hemisphere. Although there is currently no vaccine against malaria, several different anti-malarial drugs can provide protection when you travel. Start taking the drugs up to a week before you leave. You may need to keep taking them for up to four weeks after you return, depending on which medication you are taking.

In some countries, food and drinks can be contaminated with pathogens. If this is a problem in an area you're visiting, follow these tips:

◆ Eat food that is hot and cooked through, peel fruit before you eat it, drink only bottled water or carbonated drinks, and brush your teeth and mix infant formula with bottled water.

◆ Avoid raw seafood and salads, food from street vendors, unpasteurized milk and cheese, and ice.

You also might need to take additional safety precautions in some countries, such as using DEET-based (DEET is the active ingredient that repels mosquito and tick bites) or other insect repellents, using mosquito nets when you sleep, or avoiding freshwater swimming.

It's smart to pack a traveler's first aid kit and keep it with you at all times when you travel. Your kit should include pain relievers, antiseptic ointment, bandages, insect repellent, sunscreen, alcohol-based hand rubs, medicines for stomach problems and diarrhea, cold medicine, allergy medicine, hydrocortisone cream, moleskin, tweezers, scissors, nail clippers, a pocket knife, and a thermometer. Ask your doctor whether you should bring anything else in your kit to help treat specific medical problems.

Health Advisory

If you need medical help when you are traveling abroad, the United States Embassy (usually located in the host country's capital) or the United States Consulate (the embassy's "branch offices," sometimes located in other cities in the host country) can help you locate a nearby health-care provider or hospital. You can look up these agencies online at http://usembassy.gov.

After you return from your trip, be aware of your health and your family's health, especially if you traveled to an area where malaria is common. Talk to your doctor right away if you develop a fever or flulike symptoms within a year of your trip. If you develop any other worrisome medical problems after traveling abroad, talk to your doctor as well. Be sure to mention that you traveled recently, and tell him or her where you went.

Common Vaccinations by Region

If you are up to date on all your routine vaccinations, the additional vaccinations you'll need depend largely on where you are traveling to because certain vaccine-preventable infectious diseases are especially common in some areas of the world.

Typhoid

Typhoid fever is a common problem in many countries and can be a threat to travelers in South Asia, Asia (including Pakistan and India), the Caribbean, Central America (including Mexico), South America, and Africa.

You will likely need a typhoid vaccination if you will be spending more than a month in rural areas and small cities in regions where typhoid is common. You may also need a typhoid vaccination if you plan to do adventure travel abroad and will be eating and drinking far from urban centers.

Typhoid fever is caused by a type of salmonella bacteria and is spread through food or drinks contaminated with infected human feces. The salmonella bacteria that cause typhoid fever in other countries cause more dangerous infections than the salmonella bacteria that sometimes infect the United States' food supply.

The main symptom of typhoid fever is a high fever (up to 104°F), although you can also develop a headache, rash, enlarged spleen, and other problems. In rare cases, typhoid can be fatal. There are two typhoid vaccines available: a live, attenuated vaccine (licensed in 1989) and an inactivated vaccine (licensed in 1994).

Health Advisory

Be sure to tell your doctor if you have had a life-threatening reaction to a dose of a vaccine or to a vaccine ingredient. You might not be able to receive some vaccinations. If you are somewhat or very ill with an acute (short-term) illness on the day you are scheduled to receive a vaccination, tell your doctor as well. The vaccination might be postponed until you feel better.

The live vaccine is given orally as a series of four capsules, with a 48-hour gap between each pill. The pills need to be refrigerated and taken with a cool drink an hour before a meal. The last pill should be taken at least one week before your trip to guarantee maximum immunity to typhoid. The live vaccine is only approved for people six years old and older, and it provides immunity to typhoid for five years.

The inactivated vaccine is given as one injection. This vaccine should be given at least two weeks before your trip to ensure maximum immunity. The inactivated vaccine is approved for children ages two and older, and it provides immunity to typhoid for two years.

After vaccination with the live or inactivated typhoid vaccine, you might have a fever or headache. After vaccination with the inactivated vaccine, you might have swelling at the injection site. On rare occasions, the live vaccine (capsules) causes side effects such as stomach pain, vomiting, or a rash.

Neither vaccine is recommended for pregnant women, because the effects of receiving the vaccine during pregnancy are unknown. The live vaccine should not be given to people with weakened immune systems due to a disease or medical treatment. You should not receive the live vaccine within 24 hours of taking some types of antibiotics.

Because the typhoid vaccine is 50 to 80 percent effective at preventing typhoid, vaccination does not guarantee immunity to it. If you travel in areas where typhoid is common, it's important to be careful about what you eat and drink, as noted earlier in this chapter, even if you have been vaccinated against typhoid.

Yellow Fever

Yellow fever is a much less common threat to travelers, but proof of vaccination might be required to enter certain countries. It occurs in parts of Africa (except South Africa) and tropical South America.

Yellow fever is a viral infection spread by mosquito bites. Mosquitoes act as a *vector* for the virus,

def•i•ni•tion

Some diseases are spread to humans by another organism, such as a mosquito or a tick. These disease carriers are called **vectors**.

which cannot be spread from person to person. The virus can cause liver inflammation and bleeding problems. It is called yellow fever because the liver inflammation can lead to jaundice, or yellowing of the skin. The virus can also cause flulike symptoms such as muscle aches, fever, and chills. About 20 percent of people who catch yellow fever die of the disease due to liver damage and bleeding. Yellow fever epidemics are seasonal, with epidemics more common at certain times of the year.

Vaccinating Facts
If a yellow fever vaccination is required to enter a country, you must provide an International Certificate of Vaccination or Prophylaxis (ICVP) that proves you have been vaccinated. The certificate is valid for 10 years. You can get the vaccination and certificate at a yellow fever vaccination clinic. To find one near you, visit wwwn.cdc.gov/travel/yellow-fever-vaccination-clinics-search.aspx.

The yellow fever vaccine, which was created in the 1930s, is a live vaccine that is given by injection. International regulations require proof of yellow fever vaccination to enter or travel between certain countries. You must provide official documentation of a yellow fever vaccination or provide a medical waiver from your doctor explaining why you can't have the vaccination (such as an immune system disorder or pregnancy). Some countries with yellow fever vaccination requirements allow waivers for children under one year old. If you have a medical waiver letter, however, you still might not be allowed to enter the country.

One injection of the yellow fever vaccine provides immunity to the disease for 10 years. Children nine months old and older can receive the vaccine. A child might be able to receive a yellow fever vaccine if he or she is as young as six months of age if the vaccination is deemed necessary. Serious side effects from the vaccination are more common in young infants, and infection with yellow fever is also more likely to be serious in infants and children. The vaccination should be received at least 10 days before travel.

Side effects after the vaccination include flulike symptoms such as a headache or low fever. A rash, hives, and other more serious reactions are rare. Rarely, yellow fever–like illness or neurological problems, including Guillain-Barré Syndrome (GBS), have occurred after yellow fever vaccination. Serious side effects might be more common in people older than 60.

The yellow fever vaccine should not be given to pregnant or nursing women unless absolutely necessary. People with weakened immune systems due to disease or medical treatments, a history of disease of the thymus, a severe allergy to eggs or chicken, and infants under six months old should not receive this live vaccine. Also, tell your doctor if you have a severe allergy to gelatin.

Because yellow fever is spread by mosquitoes that come out at night, when traveling in an area where it's common, use mosquito netting on your bed, wear mosquito repellent that contains DEET, and wear long-sleeved shirts and pants to prevent bites. Avoid going outside at night, and remain inside screened-in areas when going outside is necessary.

Japanese Encephalitis

Japanese encephalitis can be a problem in South and Southeast Asia and occurs in seasonal outbreaks. It is a viral disease spread by mosquitoes and is not spread from person to person. The virus can cause brain inflammation, fever, nausea, and other problems. The virus is very dangerous to humans, and children are especially vulnerable to it. Twenty-five percent of people who catch the virus die from it, and people who do survive the infection often have brain damage.

The Japanese encephalitis vaccine is an inactivated vaccine, licensed for use in the United States in 1992. Health reports indicate it will be replaced with a different, inactivated version of the vaccine in the near future.

The Japanese encephalitis vaccine is usually given in three doses over 30 days, with the second dose 7 days after the first dose, and the third dose 30 days after the first dose. You should finish the series of shots 10 days before you travel to ensure maximum immunity to the virus. If necessary, your doctor might follow an accelerated schedule, with doses 7 and 14 days after the first dose, or follow a two-dose schedule. Immunity after vaccination is believed to last two years. The vaccine is not recommended for children under one year old.

Side effects after vaccination can include pain at the injection site and flulike symptoms such as fever, chills, muscle aches, and headache. Rarely, severe allergic reactions can occur, including hives and breathing problems, after any of the doses. Neurological problems are also a rare but possible side effect of the vaccine. Pregnant women should only receive the vaccine if they are at high risk of catching Japanese encephalitis. Tell your doctor if you have a severe allergy to gelatin or wasp stings.

Because this vaccination is not 100 percent effective, it is important to take steps to avoid mosquitoes, especially at night, in areas where Japanese encephalitis is a problem. As with yellow fever, mosquito netting, DEET-based insect repellent, and wearing long-sleeved shirts and long pants can help protect you from mosquito bites.

> **Vaccinating Facts**
>
> Japanese encephalitis is common in rural areas of Asia where there are many rice fields. Mosquitoes that spread Japanese encephalitis breed in flooded rice fields and pick up the virus by biting infected wild birds that wade in the fields and local infected domesticated pigs. Then the mosquitoes pass the virus from animals to humans.

Even if you take these precautions, however, you might need the vaccine if you spend more than a month in an area where Japanese encephalitis is a problem, or if you are visiting a rural area in the region where it is common. You should also be vaccinated if you plan to be outside often during your travels.

Rabies

Rabies is a problem on almost every continent. It can be a special threat to travelers in Africa, Central and South America, and Asia. As discussed in Chapter 9, it is a fatal viral disease that animals can give to humans through their saliva, causing hallucinations, seizures, and other symptoms. Outside the United States, the disease is most often transmitted by infected dogs. Other animals such as bats, raccoons, foxes, skunks, and cats also give rabies to humans.

In the United States, a person exposed to rabies (or who might have been exposed to rabies) receives a series of post-exposure shots during the virus's incubation period to prevent a rabies infection. Travelers, however, can receive a pre-exposure rabies vaccination.

A pre-exposure rabies vaccination does not prevent rabies if you are bitten during your travels, but it reduces the number of shots you will need to treat rabies after a bite. If you will be far from medical care during your travels, the pre-exposure vaccination can provide some protection until you can get adequate treatment. If you are traveling with children to an area where rabies is common, they may need a pre-exposure rabies vaccination as well because children can often be tempted to play with animals. See Chapter 9 for specifics on rabies vaccine dosing and side effects.

> **Health Advisory**
>
> To decrease the chance of catching rabies when you're traveling, avoid contact with wild animals. Avoid touching household pets as well, because they might not be vaccinated against rabies. Also, when traveling, keep children away from animals.

Hepatitis A Vaccination

The hepatitis A virus is a problem worldwide, and no areas of the world are more or less prone to having it. It can be spread through contaminated food or water, and it is a very common infection among travelers.

As discussed in Chapter 5, hepatitis A affects the liver, causing diarrhea, severe stomach pain, jaundice, fever, and other symptoms, and often requires hospitalization. In some cases, infection with hepatitis A can be fatal. The hepatitis A vaccination requires two doses. The second dose should be at least six months after the first dose. If you are not vaccinated against hepatitis A and you are traveling soon, however, the first dose can provide good protection against hepatitis A if you receive it any time before you leave. The second dose extends this immunity for many years. Depending on your age and health, you also might receive a dose of hepatitis A immune globulin with or instead of a vaccination to ensure short-term protection. See Chapter 4 for more specifics on hepatitis A dosing and side effects.

A combination vaccine containing vaccines against hepatitis A and hepatitis B is also available for people 18 years old and over. It can be given on an accelerated three-dose schedule over 21 days to provide protection for travelers, with a booster shot a year later.

> **Health Advisory** _____
>
> Many adults today have not received a routine hepatitis B vaccine, which was added to the childhood vaccination schedule in the 1980s. Hepatitis B can cause liver damage or even be fatal in some cases. If you have not been vaccinated against hepatitis B and you plan to travel to a country where hepatitis B is common, such as parts of Africa and Asia, it's a good idea to get vaccinated against hepatitis B.

All travelers should make sure they are up to date on their standard recommended vaccinations, such as the measles, mumps, and rubella (MMR) vaccine. Travelers might also need these additional vaccines:

Vaccinations for Travelers

Vaccine	Prevents	Doses	Vaccinate By: *
Typhoid	Typhoid fever	Oral: 4 capsules	Over 6 days, 1 week before travel
		Injected: One dose	2 weeks before travel
Yellow fever ***	Yellow fever	One dose	10 days before travel
Japanese encephalitis	JE	Three doses: second dose 7 days after first; third dose 30 days after first travel	10 days before travel

Vaccine	Prevents	Doses	Vaccinate By: *
Rabies (prophylactic)	Rabies	Three doses: second dose 7 days after first; third dose 21 or 28 days after first **	As soon as possible after contact
Hepatitis A	Hepatitis A	Two doses 6 months apart	6 months before travel

Note: A one-dose meningococcal vaccine might be required for travel to Saudi Arabia during certain times of the year.
* If time is limited, your health-care provider might follow an accelerated vaccination schedule.
** If you are exposed to rabies after prophylactic vaccination, you need two more doses of the vaccine, 3 days apart. In the near future, prophylactic rabies vaccination might require four doses rather than five doses.
*** Proof of this vaccination is required to enter certain countries.

The Least You Need to Know

- The CDC website is a valuable resource for learning about what vaccinations are needed when traveling to different parts of the world.

- Some vaccinations are legally required to enter certain countries, but most are just recommended.

- See your doctor at least one month before traveling to be able to get any necessary vaccinations.

- Be advised of what is safe and not safe to eat and drink when traveling in areas outside the United States.

- Protection from animals and insects when traveling is important because they can carry and pass on certain diseases.

Chapter 11

Vaccines on the Horizon

In This Chapter

- ◆ What scientific and social obstacles researchers face in developing new vaccines

- ◆ Why vaccines are important even if there are other treatments for a disease

- ◆ Three diseases that are most in need of effective vaccines

- ◆ How vaccines can help control noninfectious diseases such as cancer

Vaccines against common infectious diseases save both lives and health-care costs, and new vaccines are an important public health investment. Countries with limited health-care resources can benefit the most from vaccines against common, often deadly diseases such as malaria. Drug-resistant strains of common diseases make the need for new vaccines especially acute. Vaccines aren't just useful for preventing infections. Vaccine researchers are working on vaccines that teach the immune system to control a noninfectious disease even after it develops. These vaccines have the potential to expand treatment options for some serious diseases such as cancer. As vaccine science advances, the number of diseases that vaccines might be able to treat also grows.

Challenges to Creating New Vaccines

While modern vaccines have saved the lives of millions of people around the world, especially children, infectious diseases are still a leading cause of death worldwide. There are still no vaccines available for some diseases, and the vaccines currently available for some others, such as tuberculosis, provide only limited protection from the disease.

There are barriers to creating and distributing new vaccines for many common infectious diseases. Funding and distribution issues are two big challenges, which are covered in detail in Chapter 15. Another big challenge to creating new vaccines is that many of the pathogens that cause disease are very complex—to say the least—and researchers don't yet completely understand how they affect the immune system. It is difficult to create an effective vaccine until researchers know exactly how these pathogens cause certain diseases.

Researchers continue to study, test, and develop new vaccines despite the complexities and challenges. New vaccines under development have enormous potential to prevent suffering and death from infectious diseases worldwide, especially among children.

New Vaccine Techniques

Recent scientific advances have provided many new tools to create and administer vaccines. The standard vaccines received today include live, attenuated vaccines (which are effective, but can be dangerous for people with weakened immune systems); inactivated vaccines (which are slightly less effective, but safe for people with weakened immune systems); and toxoid vaccines (which are made from bacterial toxins). Conjugate vaccines, often used for children, link a piece of a bacterium to a biological "carrier" that helps the immune system recognize and respond to the vaccine.

Some vaccines, called subunit vaccines, use just a pathogen's antigen(s) or part of a pathogen's antigen to trigger an immune response in your body. Both the hepatitis B vaccine and the human papillomavirus (HPV) vaccine are subunit vaccines that create immunity using a piece of a virus, rather than the whole weakened or inactivated virus. Subunit vaccines are very effective at creating immunity, and they are safer for people with weakened immune systems than live, attenuated vaccines.

The concept of deoxyribonucleic acid (DNA) vaccines takes this idea one step further. Instead of using an antigen—or a part of one—to create immunity, DNA vaccines contain a piece of genetic code for an antigen. A person's cells then use the code—which has been genetically altered so that it cannot cause disease—to create the antigen, and the immune system responds to the antigen to create immunity. There are no DNA vaccines available yet, but it is considered a promising area of vaccine research.

Sometimes a subunit vaccine or a DNA vaccine is combined with a biological vector, or carrier, such as a harmless virus. Because the vaccine is combined with a vector, it is called a recombinant vaccine. This vector delivers the piece of the antigen, or code for the antigen, to the cells.

Some researchers are looking into using new types of adjuvants to improve how well vaccines work. Adjuvants are vaccine additives that help your body recognize and respond to the vaccine, making the vaccine more effective. Vaccines that contain adjuvants may also contain smaller amounts of the modified pathogen than those without adjuvants. This can save time and money when producing vaccines.

Three Critical New Vaccines

Although vaccines for many different diseases are currently being researched and developed, malaria, tuberculosis, and HIV/AIDS are receiving special attention in vaccine research. These three diseases are both widespread and devastating worldwide. Fortunately, researchers are closing in on new vaccines for each of these diseases.

Health Advisory

Each year, about 330 million people are infected with malaria worldwide, and 1 million people die of the disease, according to the World Health Organization. Worldwide, about 2 billion people are infected with tuberculosis, and about 33 million people are infected with HIV.

The Malaria Vaccine

Malaria is an infectious disease caused by a parasite. One of the four types of malaria parasites causes more serious illness than the others. A malaria infection can cause fever and chills, sweating, fatigue, muscle pain, and headache. In some cases, malaria can lead to fatal kidney, brain, or blood problems. Sometimes, malaria symptoms don't appear until months or years after a person gets infected.

About one million people die of malaria each year, primarily in sub-Saharan Africa, yet malaria also occurs in other parts of the world such as Asia, South America, and the Middle East. Although malaria is extremely rare in the United States (most U.S. cases occur among travelers who visit areas where malaria is common), about half of the world's population lives in the areas where they can be exposed to the disease. Children under five years old are most likely to die of malaria, and infection with malaria can kill or harm a pregnant woman and her child.

Malaria does not spread through person-to-person contact. Instead, this disease is spread by certain species of mosquitoes that act as disease vectors (two of these species can be found in the United States). If a mosquito infected with a malaria parasite bites you, the parasite in the mosquito's saliva then enters your bloodstream. From there, the parasite travels to your liver, where it enters liver cells and grows. Once it has matured, the parasite breaks open the liver cells and enters your blood, where it reproduces and causes symptoms. If a mosquito bites you after the parasite has reproduced in your blood, the parasite enters the mosquito and the mosquito can then give malaria to another person.

If you travel to an area where malaria is common, oral medications can be taken to prevent it. Unfortunately, these medications are not a practical solution for people who live in areas where malaria is common. The medications are expensive and can cause side effects if they are taken for a long time. Malaria prevention programs in these areas focus on controlling mosquitoes that carry the disease. Successful strategies include using insecticide to kill mosquitoes that transmit malaria and distributing insecticide-treated nets to cover beds and provide protection from mosquito bites at night.

Vaccinating Facts
The Centers for Disease Control and Prevention (CDC) began as an organization to fight malaria in the United States. During World War II, many U.S. soldiers were exposed to malaria in their training areas in the southern United States or on the battlefield. Researchers worked to control the spread of malaria among soldiers and from soldiers to civilians (they controlled malaria by using insecticides to kill the mosquitoes that spread the disease). In the mid-1940s, the Communicable Disease Center was established to continue this work. It was later renamed the Centers for Disease Control, then the Centers for Disease Control and Prevention.

Unfortunately, the mosquitoes that transmit malaria are developing resistance to the most effective insecticides. The malaria parasite is also developing resistance to the most effective medications used to treat malaria. Furthermore, in countries where malaria is common, many people cannot afford or do not have access to medical treatment for malaria.

Because malaria is becoming more difficult to prevent and treat, there is an urgent need for an effective malaria vaccine. The vaccine would target the malaria parasite during one of its life stages, either before or when it entered the liver, when it reproduced in the blood, or when it was transmitted by a mosquito from one human to another. The most promising malaria vaccine being developed is a recombinant vaccine that combines inactivated pieces of the malaria parasite and the hepatitis B virus and targets the parasite before it reaches a person's blood to reproduce. Recent studies of this vaccine in Africa have found it about 50 percent effective in preventing malaria in children under two years old. A vaccine even 50 percent effective against malaria could save many lives as part of a malaria control program.

The Tuberculosis Vaccine

Tuberculosis is a sometimes-fatal bacterial infection that often affects the lungs (called pulmonary tuberculosis). Someone with tuberculosis might cough up mucus or blood, feel weak and feverish, have chest pain, and lose weight. Tuberculosis can also spread to other parts of the body, such as the brain, kidneys, or bones (called extrapulmonary tuberculosis).

Vaccinating Facts

In the past, tuberculosis was called consumption. Because pulmonary tuberculosis causes weight loss and other problems, the illness seemed to "consume" people and make them waste away.

def•i•ni•tion

A *latent* tuberculosis infection does not cause symptoms and is not infectious. If symptoms such as coughing do appear, the infection has become **active** and it can be passed on to other people.

Usually, a person's immune system does a good job of suppressing tuberculosis, so that they do not have symptoms when they first become infected. This is called a *latent* tuberculosis infection, which may be diagnosed with a positive skin or blood test. Instead, tuberculosis symptoms might appear months or years after infection, often when the immune system is weakened by another disease. Medications can stop a latent tuberculosis infection from becoming an *active* infection that causes symptoms. Latent tuberculosis is not contagious, but active (or symptomatic) pulmonary tuberculosis is very contagious.

Like malaria, tuberculosis is relatively rare in the United States but very common in many other countries, especially those in sub-Saharan Africa and Southeast Asia. It is also a health threat for people who travel to these areas. Worldwide, one out of every three people is infected with tuberculosis, and about two million people die of the disease each year. Children under five years old, whose immune systems are less robust than adults, are most likely to have the most serious infections. Tuberculosis is spread through the air by coughing, sneezing, or talking, when someone spends a lot of time near a person with an active infection.

Tuberculosis can be treated successfully with several months of antibiotics. Unfortunately, some of the bacteria that cause tuberculosis have become resistant to the most effective antibiotics, and this form of tuberculosis is called multidrug-resistant tuberculosis (MDR TB). These infections must be treated with a group of antibiotics that are less effective against tuberculosis, more expensive than the other antibiotics, and have more side effects. The medications to treat MDR TB also must be taken for a longer time than the more effective antibiotics—sometimes as long as two years. These less effective antibiotics don't always work because a few forms of tuberculosis (called extensively drug-resistant tuberculosis, or XDR TB) have become resistant to them as well. Therefore, treating XDR TB is extremely difficult.

Health Advisory

Drug-resistant tuberculosis can develop when patients do not take all of their prescribed antibiotics, and some tuberculosis bacteria survive and develop resistance to these antibiotics. Sometimes, patients stop taking antibiotics because they feel better and think they don't need to finish the full course of medications. In countries with inadequate health-care systems, however, it also might be hard for patients to obtain all the antibiotics needed for treatment, which contributes to the problem of drug resistance.

A live, attenuated vaccine, made from a type of tuberculosis common in cows (called bovine tuberculosis), was developed for tuberculosis in the 1920s. The vaccine, called the Bacille Calmette-Guérin (BCG) vaccine, is still widely used around the world. This vaccine is effective at preventing a life-threatening type of tuberculosis in children, but is less effective at preventing pulmonary tuberculosis in adolescents and adults.

The vaccine has other limitations as well. It can cause positive results in a tuberculosis skin test even if a person doesn't have the disease. Because the BCG vaccine is a live vaccine, people with weakened immune systems cannot receive it. Unfortunately, these are the people who would benefit greatly from it because people with weakened immune systems who are exposed to tuberculosis are more likely to develop active tuberculosis than those with healthy immune systems.

Vaccinating Facts

Since the BCG vaccine can prevent a form of childhood tuberculosis, about a hundred countries worldwide recommend the BCG vaccine for infants and children. As a result, the BCG vaccine is one of the most commonly used vaccines in the world.

In the United States, the BCG vaccine is recommended only if a child lives with someone who has untreated or untreatable tuberculosis. The BCG vaccine is not a standard childhood vaccination because tuberculosis is rare in the United States. But, because there is such a great need for a better tuberculosis vaccine in other parts of the world, researchers are currently trying many different ways to create a better vaccine. An inhaled and a new oral version of the BCG vaccine are being investigated, which might be more effective against pulmonary tuberculosis, as well as cheaper and easier to store and administer than the current injected vaccine.

Some tuberculosis vaccines being developed by researchers use a specially modified booster shot after the initial BCG vaccination to make it more effective. Other researchers are working to genetically modify the BCG vaccine by creating a DNA, subunit, or recombinant vaccine that would be safe for people with weakened immune systems. There are some researchers working on a live, attenuated vaccine made from the human tuberculosis bacteria rather than the bovine tuberculosis bacteria, which might be more effective than the BCG vaccine.

The HIV/AIDS Vaccine

Human immunodeficiency virus, or HIV, gradually destroys certain lymphocyte cells in the immune system, making the immune system weaker and weaker. Often, HIV infection causes no symptoms for many years. In fact, about 25 percent of people infected with HIV don't even know that they have it.

Several years after the initial infection, chronic problems such as diarrhea, weight loss, and swollen lymph nodes often develop as the virus continues to destroy the immune system. Once HIV has damaged the immune system badly enough that the infected person has a very low number of lymphocyte cells, and he or she develops a severe health problem such as certain types of pneumonia or cancer, the person is diagnosed with acquired immunodeficiency syndrome (AIDS). There is no cure for HIV or AIDS, although some medications can slow their progression. About one million people in the United States have HIV or AIDS; worldwide, AIDS is the fourth most common cause of death.

HIV is usually spread through contact with the blood or reproductive fluids of an infected person. A person who has unprotected anal, vaginal, or oral sex with someone infected with HIV can catch the virus. Drug users who share needles or other drug equipment with HIV-infected people are also at risk for catching the virus. An infected mother can give HIV to her fetus or newborn during pregnancy or childbirth, or by breast-feeding. Infection is generally *not* a concern if someone receives a blood product such as a blood transfusion because the United States has tested all donated blood for HIV since 1985.

 Brain Booster

HIV is spread through direct contact with certain bodily fluids. It is not spread through coughing or sneezing, sharing foods or drinks with an infected person, or touching something an infected person touched. HIV is not spread through a vector such as a mosquito or a tick either.

Today, 95 percent of new HIV cases are occurring in developing countries. In Africa, HIV/AIDS is the number one cause of death. Africa also has about 30 percent of all the tuberculosis cases worldwide. About 37,000 people have AIDS in the United States, according to the latest statistics. Because HIV damages the immune system, an HIV-infected person who lives in an area where tuberculosis is common is in danger of developing life-threatening tuberculosis. Hence, the HIV epidemic has contributed to the rise in tuberculosis rates worldwide.

HIV can be prevented by consistently practicing safe sex (always using condoms) and limiting the number of sexual partners. Injection drug users should never share needles or syringes. An HIV-infected woman who becomes pregnant should receive medications called antiretroviral drugs that can protect her child from the infection. These drugs can also help prevent serious infections in people infected with HIV, by decreasing the amount of virus in their blood.

An HIV vaccine could help stop the spread of HIV, particularly in countries where people have limited access to preventative measures and antiretroviral drugs. DNA vaccines, subunit vaccines, and recombinant vector vaccines are all being investigated as potential HIV vaccines. An HIV vaccine, however, probably could not stop the spread of

HIV/AIDS alone. In countries with high rates of HIV infection, the vaccine would be just one piece of a public health campaign to prevent HIV infections that might include safe sex education and other awareness tools.

HIV vaccine development has been very challenging for researchers. The HIV virus mutates frequently after infection, making it difficult for the body's immune system to respond adequately. To develop an effective vaccine, researchers need to better understand how the virus interacts with the immune system. In 2007, a promising vaccine that used another virus as a vector to deliver the vaccine was ineffective in human trials. Many preventative (prophylactic) and therapeutic (post-infection) vaccines are currently undergoing human trials. They could potentially prevent HIV infection or stop HIV from progressing to AIDS.

Other Infectious Disease Vaccines

Although malaria, tuberculosis, and HIV/AIDS are some of the most devastating infectious diseases in the world, vaccine research continues into other infectious diseases as well. Other current vaccine research focuses on vaccines to prevent certain hospital-acquired infections, vaccines to prevent potentially widespread outbreaks of infectious diseases, and vaccines to prevent certain infectious tropical diseases.

Some researchers are developing vaccines to prevent new and dangerous forms of influenza. For example, researchers are investigating a vaccine for avian influenza (bird flu), a flulike illness that in rare cases is spread from infected birds to people. Although it is not a threat right now, avian influenza has the potential to mutate and become a widespread, life-threatening infection in humans.

Historically, there have been periodic influenza *pandemics*, or widespread outbreaks, and there will probably be more influenza pandemics in the future (an *epidemic* is confined to a smaller area). There were three influenza pandemics in the twentieth century, in 1918–1919, 1957–1963, and 1968–1970. The 1918–1919 pandemic was the most famous influenza pandemic in modern history, caused by a very dangerous and very contagious form of the virus. During that outbreak, up to

50 million people died of influenza complications worldwide, including about 700,000 people in the United States.

A new type of influenza virus appeared in the spring of 2009, triggering concerns about a new influenza pandemic. This flu, first called "swine flu" and later renamed the 2009 H1N1 flu, contained genes from pig, bird (avian), and human influenza viruses.

def•i•ni•tion

A **pandemic** is an outbreak of an infectious disease, such as influenza, that affects a large number of people worldwide. An **epidemic,** on the other hand, is an outbreak that is not worldwide. It is an abnormal increase in the number of people who have a certain illness within a population or region.

Brain Booster

Pigs can catch influenza from other pigs, birds, or humans. Sometimes the influenza viruses that they catch mutate and recombine while they are in the pig's body, creating a new virus that can then sicken humans who have contact with pigs. If an influenza virus that is transmitted from an animal to a human mutates further, it might be passed from humans to humans, creating the potential for an influenza pandemic.

Some vaccines are being developed for tropical diseases, such as leishmaniasis, a parasitic disease spread by sand flies, and dengue fever, a viral disease spread by mosquitoes. These and other tropical illnesses cause harm and drain health-care resources in many parts of the world, making the need for their vaccines and research especially important.

Vaccines for Noninfectious Diseases

Some vaccines currently under development might be able to prevent noninfectious diseases as well. Most of these vaccines are therapeutic, which means they are given after the diagnosis of a disease. They are used to stop or slow the progression of the disease.

Cancer Vaccines

When cancer develops, a patient usually has three treatment options: surgery to remove any cancerous growths, radiation to destroy cancer cells with X-rays, and/or chemotherapy to destroy cancer cells with toxic medications. Radiation and chemotherapy treatments often kill healthy cells as well as cancerous ones, however, which can cause many difficult side effects.

Therapeutic cancer vaccines are a fourth cancer treatment option now under development. These vaccines are designed to help the immune system "see" and attack cancerous cells. Because cancer cells are normal cells that have mutated (changed), the immune system usually treats them like normal cells and does not recognize them as a danger. Cancer cells can also change their structure so that immune system cells don't respond to them. Therapeutic cancer vaccines have few side effects because they target only cancerous cells, not healthy cells. In the future, these vaccines could be used in combination with the other three treatment options to create better outcomes for cancer patients.

def•i•ni•tion

A **therapeutic cancer vaccine** is given after cancer is diagnosed in a patient. The vaccine uses weakened or modified cancer cells to help trigger an immune system response to the patient's cancer.

Two of the standard recommended vaccinations can help prevent cancer: the hepatitis B vaccine, which can prevent liver cancer, and the HPV vaccine, which can prevent cervical cancer in women. Because both hepatitis B and HPV infections sometimes lead to cancer, preventing the infection prevents the types of cancer they can cause. These vaccines, like other vaccines against infections, are prophylactic—working to prevent a disease before it occurs.

Therapeutic cancer vaccines, on the other hand, help fight cancer after it is diagnosed. These vaccines are developed like standard vaccines, but the "pathogen" used to make the vaccine is a cancer cell, not a virus or bacterium. Researchers use the patient's cancer cells or cancer cells from other patients to make these vaccines. The cells, or a piece of the cells, are weakened or modified in a laboratory. Then, they are injected back into the patient, in the hopes of triggering an immune response to the patient's cancer.

Although therapeutic vaccines are a promising area of cancer treatment, all the therapeutic cancer vaccines are still in the research stage in the United States and are not yet approved by the Food and Drug Administration (FDA) for use. Many of these vaccines, however, are going through clinical trials that cancer patients can join.

Patients must meet certain criteria to join a clinical trial, such as medical history or age requirements. When patients join a trial, they are told the risks and potential benefits of the trial. Researchers must follow special rules to protect the patients' health as much as possible while they participate.

Brain Booster

To find information on clinical trials for cancer, including cancer vaccines, go to the National Cancer Institute website at www.cancer.gov/clinicaltrials, or visit the National Institutes of Health (NIH) website, at www.clinicaltrials.gov. The NIH website also contains information on clinical trials for other vaccines under development, such as the HIV vaccine.

Vaccines for Addictions

Some vaccines currently being developed and tested in clinical trials might be used to treat or prevent certain addictions. Vaccines to prevent addiction to nicotine, cocaine, morphine, and other drugs work by triggering your body's antibodies to attach to and destroy the drug molecules. The drugs then can't cross from your blood to your brain and create an addictive "high." A vaccination to block the chemical processes that contribute to obesity has been studied in animal trials as well.

Vaccines for Neurological Conditions

Researchers are also investigating vaccines that could stop or slow the progression of Alzheimer's disease, a fatal neurological disorder that causes memory loss, dementia, and other problems. This disease is currently one of the top causes of death in the United States. Alzheimer's vaccines tested on animals and humans have had mixed results, and a drug that contains antibodies to substances that contribute to Alzheimer's is now being tested on humans.

Both prophylactic and therapeutic vaccines for multiple sclerosis (MS), another progressive neurological disease, are also being investigated in animal and human trials.

The Least You Need to Know

◆ Developing new vaccines is a lengthy and costly process, and effective distribution is often an inhibitor.

◆ Malaria and tuberculosis are very common diseases in parts of the world outside of the United States, making the need for these vaccines especially acute.

◆ An HIV/AIDS vaccine has been especially difficult to create due to the nature of the disease.

◆ Some vaccines under development are geared toward noninfectious diseases such as cancer and Alzheimer's disease.

Part **4**

Vaccination Controversies

You might have heard that vaccines can cause chronic illnesses and autism, and that some vaccines are made from aborted fetal cells. This part explains some of the controversies surrounding vaccines. You will also learn why vaccines sometimes don't work, what your legal rights are if a vaccine harms you, why there are periodic vaccine shortages, and what the current funding challenges are for vaccines.

Chapter 12

Do Vaccines Cause Medical Problems?

In This Chapter

- ◆ How the debate about autism and the MMR vaccination began

- ◆ What researchers now think about MMR and autism

- ◆ Other medical concerns some people have about vaccines

- ◆ Why vaccines contain certain ingredients

Vaccination has been extremely successful at preventing certain diseases, especially diseases that can harm children. Vaccine-preventable diseases such as diphtheria, measles, and *Haemophilus influenzae* type b (Hib) are now extremely rare in the United States. Some people wonder, however, whether antigens and other vaccine ingredients can cause other diseases, especially diseases common in childhood. You might have heard that vaccines cause autism, sudden infant death syndrome (SIDS), asthma, multiple sclerosis (MS), and other serious medical problems.

Are these claims true? Researchers have investigated all of them, and have not found evidence of a link between vaccinations and serious medical problems such as autism and asthma. Very rarely, a person's immune system might respond poorly to a vaccine, causing an illness (this topic is covered more in Chapter 14). But there is no evidence that receiving one or more vaccines can put you or your children at increased risk for developing a chronic illness.

Understanding Cause and Effect

When your child becomes seriously ill, you want to know why he or she became sick. If something happened to your child just before becoming ill, you might think that event caused the illness. Sometimes this reasoning is true. If your child has an asthma attack when pollen counts are high in your area, for example, the pollen might have triggered the attack. If your child's asthma worsens after she sprains her ankle, however, the asthma is not related to the sprain. The two events happened around the same time, but one did not cause the other.

What if your child develops a serious illness after receiving a vaccination? You might think that the vaccination caused the illness. Most likely, however, this is not true. Young children frequently become ill because their immune systems are exposed to different viruses and other pathogens. Colds, ear infections, rashes, and other problems are common in young children. Some children develop more serious medical problems in childhood as well.

Young children are also vaccinated against many different diseases by the time they turn two. Almost every child in the United States receives some or all of his or her recommended childhood vaccines. In the first two years of life, a child will visit the health-care provider at least eight times to receive vaccinations and get checkups. It's likely that a child will receive a vaccination around the time he or she develops a cold, an ear infection, or a more serious health problem. Just because an illness happened around the time that a child was vaccinated, however, does not mean that the vaccine caused the illness.

Vaccines and Autism

Over the past decade, a possible link between vaccination and autism has received enormous attention from both the media and researchers. The debate began with a small study published in a medical journal in 1998 that suggested that the live, weakened viruses in the measles, mumps, and rubella (MMR) vaccine might cause autism in children. Other people, concerned about vaccine ingredients (such as the mercury used in a vaccine preservative), have blamed vaccine ingredients for autism as well as other medical problems.

This debate has been complicated by a number of factors. First, parents and health-care providers often notice the symptoms of autism when a child is less than two years old, often around the time that the child receives a vaccination. The first dose of the MMR vaccination, for example, is given to children when they are 12 to 15 months old. If a young child develops autism, it may seem like the vaccination caused the problem if symptoms happened to occur around the time of a vaccination.

Second, many of the concerns about vaccines and disease have been raised by people outside the scientific community. Although concerns about a link between the type or number of vaccinations and autism have been disproved by scientific studies, some people do not believe the studies. Sometimes they misunderstand the research or believe that researchers have political or financial motivations. As a result, they refuse or limit the number of vaccinations their children receive.

What Is Autism?

To understand the debate about vaccinations and autism, you first need to understand what autism is and why it is such a concern today.

Autism is one type of developmental disorder within a group of related problems called Autism Spectrum Disorders (ASDs) or Pervasive Developmental Disorders (PDDs). Children with autism usually have problems with communication, socialization, and behavior. A child with autism might not understand nonverbal cues, such as looking in the direction someone points, or might not respond when spoken to. The child also might have trouble understanding facial expressions, or interpreting someone's tone of voice. The child might not be able to tell the difference between a smile and a harsh word from a parent. Behaviors such as repetitive head-banging or obsession with a topic or task are also common in children with autism.

Vaccinating Facts

The word autism was coined by the Swiss psychiatrist Eugen Bleuler in the early 1900s. Bleuler based the word on the Greek word *autos*, meaning "self," to show that people with autism can seem absorbed in themselves and disconnected from the world around them. Bleuler used the word autism to describe some symptoms of schizophrenia. In 1943, Leo Kanner, an Austrian doctor and psychiatrist, used the word autism to describe certain types of socially withdrawn children. Eventually, autism was seen as its own disorder, unrelated to schizophrenia.

Sometimes, symptoms of autism are present at birth. A child with autism might not reach certain developmental milestones, such as babbling and pointing at objects by 12 months old. In other cases, a child who is developing normally starts to lose certain skills or change his behavior. For example, the child might start forgetting words he or she has already learned or become withdrawn. The symptoms of autism vary with each child, who can be mildly, moderately, or severely impaired by autism. Some children with mild autism have minor symptoms and can grow up to lead normal lives.

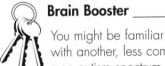

Brain Booster

You might be familiar with another, less common autism spectrum disorder called Asperger's syndrome. Children with Asperger's syndrome can communicate well verbally, but they have trouble understanding how to interact with other people in social situations and controlling their behavior.

Although autism can't be cured, it can be treated. Treatments for autism might include therapy to learn better communication, behavioral, and social skills, and medications to control anxiety and other problems.

There is no test that can prove that a person has autism. Instead, health-care providers often suggest an evaluation for autism if parents, teachers, and caregivers have noticed autism-like behavior in a child. A pediatric neurologist, psychologist, speech therapist, and other experts might observe the child and talk to the parents about the child's behavior. Evaluation should also include a hearing test because the child's behavior could be caused by a hearing problem rather than autism.

In the United States, the Centers for Disease Control and Prevention (CDC) estimates that about 1 in 150 children have autism, and autism rates appear to be increasing. Because autism can be difficult to diagnose, however, researchers do not know whether rates have truly increased or whether it is simply being diagnosed more often now than in the past.

 Brain Booster

Autism is four times more common in boys than in girls.

The definition of autism has changed over the years, making it difficult to compare today's autism rates with past autism rates. The American Psychiatric Association uses a list of symptoms in the *Diagnostic and Statistical Manual* (DSM) as a guideline to diagnose autism. The DSM did not list autism as a diagnosis until 1980, and the DSM's definition of autism has changed over the years to include a wider range of symptoms in revisions since 1980.

The causes of autism are still unknown. Many researchers believe that some children are genetically inclined toward developing autism, but don't develop it unless there is an environmental "trigger," such as a viral infection. Some people have suggested that vaccines might be this trigger.

A lot of scientific evidence indicates that autism has a genetic cause. For example, history of autism-like behaviors or emotional disorders in a family might increase the chances that a child will develop autism. If one child has autism, his or her sibling is at increased risk for developing the disorder as well. In studies of twins published in medical and psychiatric journals, if one identical twin has autism, the other twin (who has the same genes) has a much higher chance of developing autism than a fraternal twin would (a fraternal twin shares far less genetic material with his or her sibling).

Brain Booster

The Autism Coordinating Committee coordinates federal services for children with autism and their families. The committee works with the Department of Health and Human Services, the Centers for Medicare and Medicaid Services, the Office on Disability, and the Department of Education, among other organizations.

Whatever the cause, autism can be an enormous challenge for a family. Children with autism often require intensive interventional treatment to help them develop as normally as possible. They might become upset if their daily routine changes, not want to be touched or spoken to, and they might have trouble communicating what they need.

The Wakefield Study

In 1998, an English gastroenterologist named Andrew Wakefield and 12 colleagues published a study on gastrointestinal disease and autism in the British medical journal *The Lancet.* The study looked at 12 children, ages 3 to 10, who developed normally at first but then developed both intestinal problems and behavioral problems. Nine of the children were diagnosed with autism. The parents of eight of the children in the study said that behavioral symptoms began after their child received a measles, mumps, and rubella (MMR) vaccination.

As you know by now, the MMR vaccine is a live, attenuated vaccine. Wakefield and his colleagues came up with a *hypothesis*, or theory, that the weakened viruses included in the MMR vaccine might be a trigger for a disease that causes both intestinal and developmental problems. They thought that the intestinal problems might cause damaging substances to enter the bloodstream from the intestines. From there, the substances might reach the brain, causing developmental problems such as autism.

def•i•ni•tion

A **hypothesis** is a theory about a scientific process or an illness that a researcher tries to either prove or disprove through laboratory research and data analysis.

The Wakefield study caught the attention of the media and triggered an international debate about vaccines and autism. Along with questions about the MMR vaccine, some people questioned the safety of vaccine ingredients (such as the preservative thimerosal) and the number of vaccines given to young children (issues addressed later in this chapter). As a result of the Wakefield study, some parents refused the MMR vaccination for their children.

In the years following the Wakefield study, Britain's MMR vaccination rates dropped by about 20 percent, and measles outbreaks occurred in both Britain and the United States. Measles is extremely contagious, and measles outbreaks have occurred here when an unvaccinated person has caught the virus in another country and then entered the United States. In a study of measles cases in Colorado from 1987 to 1998, unvaccinated people were 22 times more likely to catch measles than those who were vaccinated. In 2008, over 100 Americans caught measles. Most of them were unvaccinated, either by choice or circumstance.

Questioning Wakefield

Many studies have been done on vaccines and autism since 1998. Over the years since Wakefield's study, studies of larger populations of children with autism, which provided more accurate data than studies of just 12 people, did not find evidence that the MMR vaccine causes autism.

For example, a 2002 study of over 500,000 Danish children, published in *The New England Journal of Medicine*, found that MMR-vaccinated children had the same rates of autism and ASDs as those who were not vaccinated. A 2004 review by the Immunization Safety Committee of the Institute of Medicine (IOM), an independent agency that advises the federal government on science policy,

> **Brain Booster**
>
> The Institute of Medicine (IOM), a division of the National Academy of Sciences, was created in 1970 to advise the U.S. government and the public about medicine and science. Members of the IOM, who are experts in their fields, create reports, studies, and policy statements about medicine, usually at the request of the federal government.

reached similar conclusions. The committee reviewed studies and found no evidence that the MMR causes autism.

Wakefield himself was also investigated for breaches of medical ethics. In 2005, England's medical association filed charges against him, claiming that he had improperly recruited patients and had conducted unapproved invasive tests (such as spinal taps) on children, among other charges. A reporter in London found evidence that Wakefield was funded in part by a personal injury lawyer, who represented some of the children in the study, a connection that Wakefield later admitted. Because their families were looking for evidence that the MMR vaccination had caused their child's autism, Wakefield's 1998 study was considered biased due to a conflict of interest.

Most of the original authors of the Wakefield study later retracted their opinions because they were concerned about the allegations against Wakefield and the study's impact on vaccination rates. Wakefield did not retract the study and now works with autistic patients in the United States.

Mercury

Although a possible link between weakened vaccine viruses and autism has been disproved, some people believe that other vaccine ingredients might cause autism. In particular, they have raised questions about thimerosal, a mercury-containing preservative that has been used to prevent the growth of contaminants such as bacteria in vaccines since the 1930s. Thimerosal is also used as a preservative in some other medical and health products, such as contact lens solutions.

Fish and shellfish that live in mercury-polluted waters absorb the mercury from the food they eat. If people eat the fish, a type of mercury called methyl mercury can build up in their bodies as well. If enough mercury builds up in your body, you can develop problems walking, hearing, talking, and concentrating, as well as muscle tremors.

Some of these symptoms may appear similar to the signs of autism, although mercury poisoning is not the same as autism. As the number of childhood vaccines has increased over the years, each child's exposure to thimerosal, which contains a different type of mercury called ethyl mercury, through vaccination has also increased. Parents, activists, and some researchers raised questions about whether the amount of thimerosal in current childhood vaccines could cause autism.

Brain Booster

The preservative thimerosal is made of ethyl mercury, which has a different chemical composition than the type of mercury sometimes found in fish (called methyl mercury). Ethyl mercury is less toxic than methyl mercury, and is less likely to build up to harmful levels in a child's body. There have been more studies of methyl mercury than ethyl mercury, however. As a result, thimerosal exposure guidelines are based on data about the more potent methyl mercury.

The Food and Drug Administration (FDA) looked at the amount of ethyl mercury in childhood vaccines and found that the amount of thimerosal children were exposed to through vaccinations exceeded the amount of more toxic methyl mercury considered safe to eat in fish. In 1999, in response to both public concern and in an effort to decrease mercury exposure in young children, the American Academy of Pediatrics and other health organizations asked vaccine manufacturers to remove thimerosal from vaccines given to children. Vaccine manufacturers reformulated their vaccines to remove thimerosal from almost all vaccines given to children under seven years old. Some versions of the inactivated influenza vaccine (the "flu shot") still use thimerosal as a preservative. Since 2001, however, all the other childhood vaccines now either do not contain thimerosal or contain only trace amounts of it.

This move did not affect autism rates in the United States. The IOM's Immunization Safety Committee report on autism and vaccines in 2004 found no evidence that the thimerosal in vaccines caused autism. A study of statewide autism rates in California from 1995 to 2007, published in the Archives of General Psychiatry in 2008, also found that the number of children who developed autism did not decline after thimerosal was removed from childhood vaccines.

Next Steps

Several children who developed autism after an MMR vaccination recently had their cases heard in a special vaccine court (more about the vaccine court in Chapter 14). The court reviewed almost 1,000 medical articles and considered extensive expert testimony from both sides. In early 2009, the court ruled that neither the weakened viruses in the vaccine nor other vaccine ingredients such as thimerosal had caused the children's autism.

Some people still believe that some other part of vaccines might cause autism. Most researchers do not believe that vaccines cause autism and believe that research funds and studies should now focus on other possible causes, such as the role of genetics in autism.

The CDC is currently conducting a five-year Study to Explore Early Development (SEED), designed to learn more about developmental disorders such as autistic spectrum disorders. The study includes almost 3,000 children and their families from across the country. The study will look at the impact of genetics, family history, hormones, lifestyle, environment, and other factors as they relate to developmental disorders. This research might lead to treatments that could cure autism or improve the lives of children with autism and their families.

> **Brain Booster**
>
> You can learn more about the CDC's ongoing SEED study of autism and other developmental disorders on the CDC website at www.cdc.gov/ncbddd/autism/seed.htm.

Links to Other Diseases

Because many vaccines have been added to the immunization schedule in the past 30 years, infants and children receive more vaccines now than their parents did. Some parents whose children have developed health problems believe that certain vaccines, or the increased number of vaccines, caused the health problems. Some researchers have also developed hypotheses about links between certain vaccines and certain illnesses. They have examined these theories to learn more about a disease, learn more about a vaccine, or learn more about how the immune system works.

Researchers have not found evidence that the vaccines currently recommended for children and adults cause serious health problems. Despite that fact, you might have heard of possible links between the following illnesses and vaccinations.

Sudden Infant Death Syndrome (SIDS) and the diphtheria, tetanus, and acellular pertussis (DTaP) vaccination: SIDS is the sudden, unexplained death of an infant under one year old. It is the most common cause of death among children in this age group. Most SIDS deaths occur when the child is two to four months old, around the time he or she receives doses of several vaccines, including the DTaP vaccine.

These deaths often occur during sleep and might be caused by a breathing problem in the infant. A national campaign to decrease SIDS, encouraging placing young children on their backs to sleep, has cut the SIDS rate by over 50 percent since 1992. While SIDS rates have fallen since 1992, the use of the DTaP vaccine has increased over that time period. The vaccine was first licensed in 1991, and the current five-dose version has been used since 1997. Because the rate of SIDS has not increased as the number of DTaP vaccinations has increased, DTaP vaccination does not seem to be linked to SIDS deaths.

Health Advisory

To protect your baby from SIDS, follow these tips from the National Institute of Child Health and Human Development's "Back to Sleep" campaign: Always put a baby to sleep lying on his or her back. Make sure the baby sleeps in a crib, bassinet, or other safe place on a firm surface, and remove any pillows, loose bedding, or soft toys. Keep the room where the baby sleeps comfortable, dress the baby lightly, and don't let anyone smoke near the baby.

In a 2003 report, the IOM's Immunization Safety Review Committee found no evidence that certain infant immunizations, including DTaP, can cause SIDS. To collect more data, a large study of DTaP and breathing and heart problems is now underway.

Asthma and vaccinations: Asthma is a very common chronic illness in children, affecting about seven million children, especially those ages five and older. Asthma is an inflammation of the airways, causing symptoms such as wheezing, coughing, and trouble breathing. Allergies, exposure to tobacco smoke, air pollution, and colds and influenza can all cause asthma, which is usually controlled with medications.

The rates of childhood asthma have been increasing in the United States since the 1980s. Some people believe that childhood vaccinations might have contributed to the asthma rates. Several large studies, however, have not found a link between asthma rates and the number or type of vaccines that children receive.

Brain Booster

Researchers are still studying why asthma rates have increased so much in all age ranges since the 1980s. Asthma is most common among African Americans, children whose parents have asthma, and people who live in urban environments (which can have worse air quality than rural and suburban environments). These factors suggest that asthma might have genetic and environmental causes.

Multiple sclerosis and the hepatitis B vaccination: Multiple sclerosis (MS) is a neurological disorder in which the immune system damages nerves in the body, causing symptoms such as trouble walking, fatigue, and numbness. About 400,000 Americans have MS. Some people have suggested that receiving the hepatitis B vaccine might increase the risk for developing multiple sclerosis. A recent study of children with and without MS, however, did not find a connection between hepatitis B vaccination and the onset of MS.

Diabetes and vaccinations: Diabetes, a disease that affects the body's ability to maintain sugar levels in the body, affects about 8 percent of all Americans, and the rate of diabetes continues to increase. Diabetes can be caused by genetics, lifestyle, and other factors. Researchers have not found evidence that vaccinations can cause diabetes.

Vaccine Ingredients

Unlike the first vaccine for smallpox, which contained only a pathogen, modern vaccines contain antigens as well as a variety of other ingredients. Several common extra ingredients a vaccine might contain today include:

♦ Preservatives to prevent contamination with bacteria and other substances.

♦ Stabilizers to keep the vaccine potent until its expiration date.

♦ Adjuvants to improve the human immune response to a vaccine.

♦ Residual materials left over from the vaccine manufacturing process.

Vaccines may contain aluminum (used as an adjuvant), formaldehyde (used as a preservative and used to create toxoid vaccines), antibiotics (used as a preservative), gelatin (used as a stabilizer), and monosodium glutamate (MSG, used as a stabilizer). Some vaccines also contain small amounts of yeast and egg protein that were used during manufacturing.

Some people believe that certain vaccine ingredients, either alone or in combination with a vaccine's weakened or inactivated pathogen, can be harmful to your health. But these ingredients are present in vaccines in very small amounts. For example, infants are exposed to much more aluminum through the environment around them than through vaccines. Formaldehyde is naturally present in the environment at higher quantities than is found in vaccines as well.

Vaccinating Facts

Adjuvants, used only in inactivated vaccines such as the DTaP vaccine, improve your immune system's response to a vaccine by acting as chemical irritants. Your immune system responds more strongly to the vaccine because your body wants to get rid of the adjuvant. Without the adjuvants in certain vaccines, the immune system might not notice the antigens, and you might not develop immunity to the disease. Adjuvants also help vaccine developers use fewer antigens in each vaccine. This decreases the chances of certain side effects and saves money in vaccine production.

In rare cases, however, a vaccine ingredient can cause an allergic reaction in a child or adult. If your child has an allergy to foods or medicines, tell your health-care provider before he or she receives a vaccination. You and your health-care provider can then discuss the risks and benefits of giving your child vaccines that might contain these substances. Often, the problem ingredient is present in such a small amount in a vaccine that it most likely will not cause an allergic reaction.

Multiple Vaccinations

Many childhood vaccines are now available as combination vaccines. The multidose DTaP vaccine and MMR vaccine are both combination vaccines. Some newer vaccines available include a DTaP and Hib combination vaccine and a DTaP, hepatitis B, and polio combination vaccine. Using a combination vaccine decreases the number of shots that your child needs to achieve immunity to vaccine-preventable diseases.

Because children are vaccinated against so many diseases when they are young, they often receive a mixture of both combination and single vaccinations in one office visit. At a child's two-month visit, for example, he or she might receive a hepatitis B, rotavirus, DTaP, Hib, pneumococcal, and polio vaccination, receiving antigens against eight different diseases at once. Some people are concerned that giving a young child many vaccines at once might damage rather than strengthen their immune system by overloading it with antigens (the part or parts of the pathogen that cause disease).

Children do receive more vaccines today than they did a generation ago. Because vaccine science has advanced over the past few decades, however, these vaccines can create immunity using far fewer antigens than vaccines used in the past. As a result, although children are receiving more vaccines than their parents did, these vaccines expose them to fewer antigens than their parents received as children. Also, infants are exposed to pathogens every day in their environment. There are bacteria on food and objects that they place in their mouths and viruses in the air they breathe. Every day, their immune system successfully fights off potential infections. The additional amount of antigens in the vaccines young children receive is small compared to the amount of pathogens that they encounter daily.

Today, vaccines protect children from many more potentially dangerous infectious diseases than their parents were protected from. The number of deaths, disabilities, and hospitalizations from diseases such as Hib, hepatitis B, and chickenpox have decreased with the introduction of new childhood vaccines.

The Least You Need to Know

◆ Medical conclusions about the MMR vaccine indicate it does not cause autism.

◆ Research shows that vaccines do not cause other diseases such as asthma or SIDS.

◆ The vaccine preservative thimerosal, which contains mercury, has been removed from most childhood vaccines.

◆ Children today receive more vaccinations but fewer antigens than generations ago.

Chapter 13

Other Questions About Vaccines

In This Chapter

- ◆ Common concerns people have about vaccines
- ◆ Religious and ethical issues related to vaccines
- ◆ Effects and consequences of not vaccinating
- ◆ How to find accurate medical data and information about vaccines

In the United States, vaccination plays an important role in protecting public health. The larger the percentage of vaccinated individuals, the safer the public is from certain infectious diseases. As vaccine-preventable diseases have decreased, however, some people have raised questions about the necessity of vaccines. Often, they have never known anyone who had serious complications from a vaccine-preventable disease, and have heard that vaccines can cause harmful side effects; therefore, they question whether vaccines are necessary, safe, or ethical.

As a result of these questions, some Americans opt out of vaccinations for themselves or their children for medical, religious, or philosophical reasons. This choice can have a direct impact on the people in the communities around them. For the majority of Americans, however, vaccinations are a safe and effective way to avoid a wide range of serious and sometimes life-threatening illnesses.

Are Vaccines Necessary?

Many vaccine-preventable diseases were extremely common in the past. Before the measles vaccine was licensed in 1963, for example, measles was so common that virtually everyone caught it before reaching adulthood. Although most measles infections did not cause serious harm, some people with measles developed pneumonia or encephalitis (brain inflammation). In the decade before the measles vaccine was licensed, about 450 U.S. citizens died from measles each year. Before vaccines for polio were developed in the 1950s, polio killed 1,000 people and paralyzed up to 20,000 people each year.

Today, however, many vaccine-preventable diseases are rare in the United States, thanks to a robust vaccination program. So, you might wonder why you or your children still need to be vaccinated against them. Haven't vaccines already done their job?

Pathogens Persist

The smallpox vaccine was used to eradicate smallpox disease worldwide, and adults and children no longer need a smallpox vaccination. It took a very long time, but the vaccination program was successful in achieving this feat. Polio is the next disease targeted for eradication, but it still occurs in the developing world. Until there are no more cases of polio worldwide, it is still a threat to anyone who is not vaccinated. An unvaccinated person who catches polio abroad could bring it to the United States and unknowingly spread the disease. Also, over the past few years, cases of measles, *Haemophilus influenzae* type b (Hib), and other vaccine-preventable diseases have occurred within the United States.

Brain Booster _____

In 2008, there were over 1,600 cases of polio worldwide. Most polio cases occur in four countries: Afghanistan, Pakistan, India, and Nigeria. Polio can spread across borders to nearby countries as well, however. In 2009, polio cases also occurred in Kenya, Sudan, Uganda, Mali, and other areas.

Today, the most common vaccine-preventable disease in the United States is influenza. Each year, about 226,000 people are hospitalized with complications of influenza, such as pneumonia, and about 36,000 people die from influenza complications. Most of the people who die are 65 years old or older—a group of people with a low influenza vaccination rate. Because the viruses that cause influenza mutate so often, people need an influenza vaccination every year to get protection from the illness.

Health Advisory _____

Some vaccine-preventable diseases can have long-term consequences even if you catch and survive the disease. Measles survivors can develop a rare, fatal form of encephalitis up to 10 years after they catch measles. Polio survivors are at risk for post-polio syndrome, with symptoms that can include muscle weakness, fatigue, and joint pain. Post-polio syndrome can occur decades after the initial polio infection.

The tetanus vaccine will always be necessary because the bacteria that cause tetanus are present in the environment all around us. Because the bacteria cannot be contained and eliminated like the smallpox virus, vaccination provides the best defense against tetanus infection. Therefore, some vaccines will always be necessary because the pathogens that cause illness probably cannot be eliminated worldwide.

Vaccines Still Save Lives

Some people believe that improvements in public health and medicine have made vaccinations unnecessary. For example, Americans now enjoy cleaner drinking water and have access to a healthier and safer food supply than they did a few generations ago. Medical advances, such as the creation of antibiotics, also provide new treatment options for diseases that were once life-threatening. So, it is true that the rates of some vaccine-preventable diseases were already decreasing due to these advances even before vaccines were created for them.

Once many vaccines were added to the vaccination schedule, however, the rates of the diseases they prevented often plummeted. Cases of varicella (chickenpox) dropped up to 86 percent in the six years after the vaccine was licensed in 1995. Furthermore, some vaccine-preventable diseases—such as meningococcal disease, which can be fatal in up to 15 percent of cases—can be difficult to treat even with modern medicines. Preventing them with vaccination is easier and safer than trying to treat them with medications.

> **Health Advisory**
>
> You might have heard it's better to develop immunity by catching and recovering from a disease (sometimes called acquired immunity) than through vaccination. Immunity acquired from an infection can be risky because every vaccine-preventable disease can be dangerous on its own or carries a risk of serious complications, such as pneumonia or encephalitis. Vaccines were created to protect people from this risk. Even if you do not become seriously ill from the disease, you could pass on the disease to someone else who might have serious complications. Some vaccines, such as the Hib vaccine, also provide better protection from a disease than you would get if you caught and recovered from the disease.

For instance, improvements in public health did not stop polio. The number of polio cases in the United States was increasing in the 1950s, reaching a record high in 1952 of 21,000 cases. After the first vaccine was licensed in 1955, polio rates began to drop steeply, with fewer than 100 cases reported annually in the United States 10 years later. Thanks to widespread vaccination, the last case of wild-virus polio in the United States occurred in 1979. The last case imported into the United States from elsewhere occurred in 1993.

Are Vaccines Somehow Linked to Abortion?

Some people question vaccinations because they believe the way a vaccine is created violates their religious or ethical beliefs. Scientific advances in the twentieth century have helped researchers create vaccines for a wide range of infectious diseases. Some people have questioned, however, whether certain techniques used to create vaccines follow the ethical principles of their religion.

Viruses used to create vaccines must be grown in a living cell as they are weakened and prepared for use in vaccines. Some of these viruses grow well in animal cells, such as the influenza virus that is grown in chicken cells. Other viruses, however, grow best in human cells. These cells are called human diploid cells.

Where do these cells come from? They originally came from the lung tissue of two fetuses aborted from different mothers in the 1960s. (These abortions were not performed specifically to collect this lung tissue, however, they would have taken place regardless.) Two different strains of *human diploid cells* were developed from these tissues, and the cells have been carefully grown in laboratories over the years to be the biological environments to grow viruses in and be tools in vaccine creation. Because these cells reproduce themselves, additional fetal tissue is not needed to add to their supply. Also, there are no plans to create a new human diploid cell strain for future vaccines, so no new tissue is needed.

> **Vaccinating Facts**
>
> Human cells are used to grow most brands of vaccines for rubella (part of the MMR vaccine), hepatitis A, varicella (chickenpox), and rabies.

def•i•ni•tion

> Fetal **human diploid cells,** derived from aborted fetuses and used to make some vaccines, contain genetic material from both parents.

A rubella infection in a pregnant woman can cause a miscarriage or birth defects. Also, a pregnant woman infected with rubella is more likely to seek out an abortion if she believes the infection will cause severe damage to her baby. In a rubella epidemic that broke out a few years before the rubella vaccine became available (in 1969), about

The cells used to create the rubella vaccine came from a fetus infected with rubella.

11,000 fetuses were miscarried or aborted. In one sense, the rubella vaccine has prevented many miscarriages and abortions triggered by rubella infection in pregnant women.

People who oppose abortion, however, have sometimes struggled to decide whether to accept vaccines made with human diploid cells. Evangelical Christians, Catholics, and others who oppose abortion sometimes refuse certain vaccinations for their children because of this connection. The Catholic Church, which opposes abortion, has stated that Catholic parents can allow these vaccines for their children because the vaccines do not contribute to current abortion rates. The Catholic Church has also said that parents have an obligation to protect others from vaccine-preventable diseases and to protect their children's health. The Catholic Church is also encouraging the development of vaccines that do not use human diploid cells.

Scientific advances might allow researchers to create new versions of these vaccines in the future, but using new techniques to create these vaccines would be expensive. At the moment, vaccine manufacturers have limited incentives to change their manufacturing processes, and newer vaccines might not be as effective at preventing diseases as the current vaccines.

Religious Diets

Orthodox Muslims and Jews who follow the dietary restrictions of their faith have also questioned vaccination. Some vaccines (and other medications) contain gelatin, which is used as a stabilizer. Gelatin is made from the bones and tissues of animals such as cows, horses, and pigs. Both Muslim and Jewish traditions forbid eating pork (meat from pigs), and other meats must be prepared according to certain rules before they can be eaten.

Some Muslim scholars believe that the gelatin used in medicine is indeed acceptable for Muslims to receive for two reasons. First, gelatin is made by boiling down the animal bones and tissues, so they believe that cooking the meat in this way breaks it down and changes it so much that it becomes acceptable for Muslims to consume. Second, the gelatin in medicine and vaccines is used for medical purposes and is not eaten as a food. Because it is not used for food, scholars believe that the gelatin in medicine and vaccines is acceptable.

Jewish scholars have a similar attitude toward the gelatin found in vaccines. If the gelatin in vaccines is not taken orally as food, it is acceptable for orthodox Jews to receive.

Vaccination Requirements and Exemptions

Before a child enters day care, preschool, or elementary school, he or she should receive all the childhood vaccinations recommended for his or her age. This helps protect the child and other children from infectious diseases when they spend time together at day care or school. Children who catch infectious diseases outside the home might also bring them home and infect other household members. School-entry vaccination requirements have helped the United States achieve very high levels of childhood vaccinations.

All the states in the United States have some vaccination requirements for children entering government-sponsored preschool programs or public or private elementary school. Although these requirements vary by state, the states generally require that a child is up to date on all the recommended childhood vaccinations. To find out what your state requires, look up your state on the National Network for Immunization Information website, at www.immunizationinfo.org/VaccineInfo/index. cfm.

Vaccinating Facts

Some states or schools require that a child receive certain vaccinations, such as the DTaP, MMR, or meningococcal vaccination, before entering high school or college in that state. State health department and requirements can be found on the Centers for Disease Control and Prevention (CDC) website, at www.cdc.gov/mmwr/international/relres. html. Because these rules apply only to children entering school, home-schooled children are not required to get their recommended vaccinations.

Although vaccinations are required for school entry, there are exemptions to vaccinations for children in special circumstances. In every U.S. state, a child can be exempted from a required vaccination if he or she has a medical condition or treatment that prevents receiving the vaccination. Almost all the states allow exemptions if the parents did not vaccinate their child because the vaccination contradicts their religious beliefs. About half the states also allow a philosophical exemption if parents disagree with a vaccination for other reasons. In states with more exemption options, more parents opt out of vaccination; as a consequence, these states have higher rates of vaccine-preventable diseases, such as pertussis. If a child receives an exemption, he or she might not be able to attend school if there is an outbreak of a vaccine-preventable disease at the school.

In other cases, some parents ask for an exemption because they think that vaccinations are unnecessary or harmful. They might believe that their child is unlikely to be exposed to a vaccine-preventable disease, or that they can boost their child's immune system with vitamins, herbs, and other alternative medicines. Some parents oppose the idea of a vaccination requirement, believing it infringes on their rights to make medical decisions for their child. These exemptions raise a number of legal and ethical issues. A parent's decision not to vaccinate a child decreases the level of herd immunity in a community, impacting public health. Unvaccinated children have the potential to catch and spread a vaccine-preventable disease. Exemptions can create tension between personal rights and community rights.

The Effects of Not Vaccinating

Although most children in the United States receive all their recommended vaccinations, for various reasons some people choose not to vaccinate themselves or their children. This decision is often seen as a personal or family choice.

Choosing not to vaccinate, however, affects people beyond yourself and your family. A small percentage of children and adults cannot receive vaccinations for medical reasons. For example, children and adults who are receiving chemotherapy treatments for cancer or who are severely allergic to a vaccine ingredient might not be able to receive all their recommended vaccinations. When everyone around them is vaccinated, these vulnerable groups are protected from vaccine-preventable diseases even if they cannot receive the vaccine themselves. Without this herd immunity, however, they might catch a vaccine-preventable disease, making their circumstances much worse.

A small percentage of people who are vaccinated against a disease do not develop immunity to it. Often, they do not know that they are not immune to a disease until they catch it. Infants who have not yet received all their vaccinations are also vulnerable to disease. Both these groups rely on herd immunity to protect them from becoming ill from vaccine-preventable diseases.

Vaccination rates for certain diseases have dropped in the past, with serious consequences. Concerns about the pertussis (whooping cough) vaccine, for example, led to a 30 to 50 percent drop in immunization rates in Japan in the 1970s. A few years later, the number of pertussis cases there had increased from about 400 a year to about 13,000 a year, and about 40 people died of the disease. During the same decade in Great Britain, low vaccination rates caused an outbreak of 100,000 pertussis cases and about 40 deaths.

Many vaccine-preventable diseases are rare in the United States, but they could return if vaccination rates drop too low. Outbreaks of diseases can occur in communities that have high numbers of families who have opted out of childhood vaccinations. For example, over 90 percent of the people who caught measles during the United States' 2008 outbreak—the largest outbreak in more than a decade—were unvaccinated. Two thirds of them were unvaccinated children whose parents chose not to vaccinate them. Vaccinating yourself and your child helps keep the rates high enough to ensure adequate protection for everyone.

Evaluating Vaccine Claims

There is a wealth of information available, particularly online, about vaccine-related illnesses and injuries, but the information is not always accurate. It's important to learn how to evaluate the medical information you read and hear.

If you find vaccine information on a website, find out who runs the website and who writes the material (look in the "About Us" section of the website). Are they qualified to write about this topic? Are they medical professionals? Is the site reviewed by a medical professional, or a group of medical professionals, to ensure it is accurate? If you have questions, is there a way to contact them? In general, a site run by a government agency (ending in .gov) or by an educational institution (ending in .edu) is most likely to contain accurate information. Many organization sites (ending in .org) also have accurate information.

> **Brain Booster**
>
> The Medical Library Association's "A User's Guide to Finding and Evaluating Health Information on the Web" provides useful tips and resources. It is available online at www.mlanet.org/resources/userguide.html.

If a website is trying to sell a product, the medical information on the site might be biased. Look around the site to find out who is responsible for the site, and why the site was created.

These health-based websites provide free, accurate information:

◆ The CDC's Vaccines & Immunizations, www.cdc.gov/vaccines/

◆ The National Network for Vaccination Information, www.immunizationinfo.org

◆ The Vaccine Education Center at the Children's Hospital of Philadelphia, www.chop.edu/consumer/jsp/division/generic.jsp?id=75697

A site making claims about vaccines should provide concrete data to back up these claims. Look at whether the site provides links to other reputable websites. Because medicine is constantly evolving, data from more recent studies is more accurate than data from older studies. By the same token, websites updated recently are probably more accurate than those updated several years ago. Many sites will, and should, list when certain information was updated.

These website evaluation skills can also help you evaluate health information from other sources, such as television programs, magazine articles, and friends and relatives. If you hear an unusual health claim, ask yourself who made that statement and how much medical expertise they have. Did they back up their statement with medical studies? Is this the most up-to-date information on the topic?

You might have heard personal stories about children who showed signs of autism or other problems around the time they received a vaccination. These stories can be very powerful, but it is important to put them in context. Where did you hear the story? Is the information accurate? Carefully designed studies have found no links between vaccinations and childhood diseases. One story does not prove that a vaccination is harmful, and it is unwise to base vaccination decisions on anecdotes. If you have concerns or questions about vaccinations, talk to your healthcare provider and/or reference trusted websites and materials.

The Least You Need to Know

- Although most vaccine-preventable diseases are now rare in the United States, vaccinations are still necessary.

- Some diseases will likely never be eliminated as smallpox was.

- Some vaccines are created using human cells collected from two abortions performed in the 1960s.

- Vaccinations are required for school entry in every state.

- Vaccination exemptions are available for medical, religious, or philosophical reasons in many states.

Chapter 14

When Vaccines Harm or Fail

In This Chapter

- ◆ How vaccines are monitored for side effects
- ◆ How and why a vaccine might not create immunity to a disease
- ◆ What systems are in place to monitor vaccine side effects and injuries
- ◆ What programs can help if a person is harmed by a vaccine

Vaccines, like other medications, are designed to help people; unfortunately, for some, they don't. Very rarely, a person's body might respond badly to a vaccine, causing a severe allergic reaction, or the vaccine might be contaminated, making a person ill. In other cases, a vaccine a person receives might not create immunity to that disease, putting that person at risk for catching the disease.

Fortunately, the government has several systems in place to monitor and address problems with vaccines. Data collected from health-care systems, health-care providers, vaccine manufacturers, and patients helps researchers find problems with vaccines. Vaccination prevents far more illnesses than it causes, and protecting everyone from vaccine problems is a good investment in public health.

Adverse Events

Vaccinations have decreased the number of vaccine-preventable illnesses that occur worldwide. But, on rare occasions, vaccines can cause problems. Vaccine-preventable illnesses have become much less common in the United States because so many people are vaccinated against them. Every vaccine, however, has some risk of causing a bad side effect. If you become ill after receiving a vaccine, you might wonder whether the vaccine caused the illness.

Any health problem that occurs after a vaccination is called an *adverse event*. An adverse event might be a side effect from the vaccination or an allergic reaction to the vaccine. Or, it might not be caused by the vaccination at all.

def•i•ni•tion

An **adverse event** is any health problem, such as a seizure or a high fever, that occurs during or after receiving medical treatment such as a medication or vaccination.

A small percentage of people who receive a vaccination will have an adverse event caused by the vaccine. Logically, the more people who are vaccinated, the more people will have these adverse events. For example, the measles component of the measles, mumps, and rubella (MMR) vaccine might cause thrombocytopenia, a temporary blood disorder, in about 1 in every 30,000 to 40,000 people. If one million people receive the MMR vaccination, about 25 to 33 of them might develop this problem. If five million people are vaccinated, five times as many people might develop thrombocytopenia. Someone could also have an allergic reaction to a vaccine. For example, if a person is severely allergic to latex, they could have an allergic reaction to a vaccine if it is stored in a latex container or is administered in a latex syringe.

On the other hand, an adverse event might be completely unrelated to a recent vaccination. Although vaccinations can cause a fever, for example, fevers can be caused by many different medical problems, ranging from influenza to cancer. If an adverse event is extremely rare—such as Guillain-Barré Syndrome (GBS), a neurological problem that can cause numbness and even paralysis—it can also be hard to figure out whether a vaccine caused it. There might be very few cases of different adverse events to study, too, creating a limited amount of data for researchers to analyze. Furthermore, if someone is taking medications for another medical condition, the medications might have caused the problem rather than the vaccine.

It's very important for researchers to learn whether a vaccine consistently causes a serious adverse event. If it does, the vaccine might be recalled and reformulated to make it safer, or its warning label changed. How can researchers tell whether a vaccine causes an adverse event? They ask four key questions:

- How many people who received the vaccine had this adverse event?

- How many people who received the vaccine did not have this adverse event?

- How many people who did not receive the vaccine had this adverse event?

- How many people who did not receive the vaccine did not have this adverse event?

By comparing data about these four groups of people, researchers can study whether a vaccine might cause an adverse event. When they make these comparisons, researchers choose groups of people who have similar traits to get the most accurate results. For example, they might compare data on adverse events in college-age men and women who did or did not receive the meningococcal vaccine as adolescents.

This type of data analysis has had a direct impact on the United States' vaccination program. For example, in 1976, an outbreak of swine flu occurred among military recruits in Fort Dix, New Jersey. Ultimately, one previously healthy recruit died from the disease. Authorities were concerned about the outbreak because they thought that the swine flu virus was related to the virus that caused the 1918–1919 influenza pandemic. A vaccine for swine flu was developed, and over 40 million Americans were vaccinated. However, researchers found that the number of GBS cases, normally about 1 to 2 for every 100,000 people, was slightly higher among people who had received the swine flu vaccination. Because researchers determined that it might be linked to increases in GBS, the 1976 swine flu vaccination program was suspended. Fortunately, the 1976 swine flu did not spread and become a pandemic. If it had become a pandemic, the slightly increased risk of GBS would likely have been offset by the lives saved by vaccination.

Health Advisory _____

Some vaccines can cause harm if received when an individual has an acute or chronic medical problem. Always tell your health-care provider whether you or your child are taking any medications, receiving or have recently received other medical treatments, and/or if you are or might be pregnant. Make sure your health-care provider knows your health history, in case you have had an illness in the past that might increase the risk for an adverse event from a vaccination.

Reactions

Vaccines can cause a range of side effects, and most of the side effects are mild. *Local* reactions, such as pain or swelling at the injection site, just affect the area where you receive the vaccination (usually your arm). A *systemic* reaction, on the other hand, causes symptoms in other parts of your body, such as fever or achiness. Local and systemic reactions from a vaccination usually do not cause long-term harm.

def•i•ni•tion _____

A **local** reaction to a vaccination occurs near the injection site, such as swelling. A **systemic** reaction affects other parts of the body, causing symptoms such as fever. An **allergic** reaction is a type of systemic reaction to a specific vaccine component, and it can be severe.

An *allergic* reaction is a special type of systemic reaction that occurs if your body is overly sensitive to a substance in the vaccine. Allergic reactions can be severe or life-threatening, causing problems such as skin reactions and difficulty breathing. These reactions are rare, occurring about one or two times in every one million doses of a vaccine.

Local and systemic reactions to vaccines are the most common reactions. For example, some vaccines given to adolescents, such as the human papillomavirus (HPV) vaccine, have been associated with fainting shortly after the injection. For unknown reasons, fainting after vaccination is more common in adolescents than in people in other age groups. Because some people who faint can fall and injure themselves, a health-care provider might recommend sitting down for 15 minutes after vaccinations.

Other vaccines can cause more serious problems on rare occasions. The tetanus and diphtheria components of the tetanus, diphtheria, and acellular pertussis (Tdap) vaccine can sometimes cause a severe local reaction of swelling and pain. This can occur in adults who already have antibodies to tetanus and diphtheria in their bodies. A more serious problem called brachial neuritis, on rare occasions, occurs after vaccinations for influenza, tetanus, and other illnesses. Brachial neuritis causes severe pain in one or both shoulders, and the pain can be long-term. This illness can also be caused by surgery, infections, and other diseases.

Several vaccines might be linked to very rare, serious diseases. The meningococcal conjugate vaccine (MCV4) has been linked to some cases of GBS that occurred shortly after vaccination. Because it is unclear whether the GBS cases were caused by the vaccination or whether they had other causes, researchers are still investigating any possible link.

After receiving the rotavirus vaccination, some children have developed Kawasaki disease, a rare disease in young children that causes inflammation of the arteries and can lead to heart problems and other complications. The fact that this disease appeared after rotavirus vaccination is thought to be coincidental, however, and unrelated to the vaccine. Researchers believe that rotavirus vaccination does not increase the risk for Kawasaki disease, which occurs on rare occasions in children in the general population. As with all vaccines, though, the rotavirus vaccine is continuously monitored for adverse events that might be linked to it.

Learn more about the potential side effects from each vaccine in the Centers for Disease Control and Prevention (CDC) vaccination website's section on side effects. It is located at www.cdc.gov/vaccines/vac-gen/side-effects.htm.

Manufacturing Issues

Sometimes the way a vaccine is manufactured can make it either harmful or ineffective. In the past, manufacturing problems sometimes actually caused the disease the vaccine was created to prevent. Today, manufacturing problems are more likely to make a vaccine ineffective rather than harmful. If there is a problem with a vaccine, it is recalled by the Food and Drug Administration's Center for Biologics Evaluation & Research (CBER). If the vaccine is recalled because it is ineffective, anyone who received the vaccine might need to be revaccinated.

Harmful Vaccines

In the first half of the twentieth century, a number of new vaccines were developed. Occasionally, however, some of these vaccines caused dangerous or fatal infections due to faulty manufacturing processes. In some cases, the vaccines were contaminated by bacteria or other substances, which then caused infections in people when they received the vaccine. These problems lead to the development and use of preservatives such as thimerosal in vaccines. In other cases, a vaccine accidentally contained a dangerously high amount of the live pathogen, which gave people the disease.

In 1929, for example, Bacille Calmette-Guérin (BCG, a vaccine for tuberculosis) was given to about 250 infants in Lubeck, Germany. It gave a quarter of the infants fatal cases of tuberculosis. A dangerous human strain of tuberculosis had been accidentally grown in the laboratory and used in the vaccine rather than the safer bovine (cow-based) strain of tuberculosis.

Also, in the United States, there were manufacturing problems with the first polio vaccine in 1955. One of the laboratories licensed to make the inactivated polio vaccines was Cutter Laboratories in Berkeley, California. Forty thousand of the children who received the Cutter vaccines developed polio, and ten of the children died. It turned out that some of the vaccines had contained a live rather than inactivated polio virus, causing polio in many vaccinated children. The Cutter vaccines were recalled, and it caused the government to set up more stringent vaccine manufacturing and testing standards.

More modern manufacturing problems have been far less dangerous to the public. In 2007, for example, two types of *Haemophilus influenzae* type b (Hib) vaccines, totaling about 1.2 million doses, were recalled by the manufacturer, Merck & Company. Merck recalled the vaccines because some of the equipment used to make the vaccines were contaminated with bacteria, yet no bacteria were found in the vaccines.

Ineffective Vaccines

Sometimes a vaccine is not effective at creating immunity because it was not properly manufactured, transported, or stored. The vaccine will not make you sick if you receive it, but it might not work. When this happens, either the manufacturer or the Food and Drug Administration (FDA) might recall the vaccine.

For example, in 2006, 3,000 doses of an adult tetanus and diphtheria (Td) vaccine were recalled by its manufacturer, Sanofi Pasteur, because the doses were not kept at the right temperature when they were shipped to health-care providers. As a result, the doses might not have been effective at creating immunity to tetanus and diphtheria. Also, two lots of an influenza vaccine made by the manufacturer Novartis were shipped at the wrong temperature in 2006, which might have made them ineffective.

> **Vaccinating Facts**
>
> Vaccines recalled by the FDA are listed online at: www.cdc.gov/vaccines/recs/recalls/default.htm.

Another potency problem occurred in an influenza vaccine for the 2008–2009 influenza season. In 2009, the manufacturer of five lots of influenza vaccine asked health-care providers to return them. The manufacturer's tests showed that the lots were effective in creating immunity to influenza viruses in late 2008, but they were less potent when they were tested in January of 2009.

Immune Response Failure

No vaccine creates immunity in 100 percent of the people who are vaccinated. There are always some people who don't develop immunity after they receive a vaccine. Their immune systems might not respond adequately enough to the antigens in the vaccine to create immunity to the disease. As a result, the vaccine does not harm them, but it does not protect them from disease, either.

Often, it is unclear whether a vaccine provides protection until there is an outbreak of a disease. During an outbreak, people who are unvaccinated against the disease are quite likely to catch the disease. But, a few vaccinated people might also catch the disease, if they didn't respond well to the vaccine.

To address this problem, some vaccines include multiple doses that increase the chances that you will develop immunity to the disease. The two-dose measles, mumps, and rubella (MMR) vaccine is structured this way, primarily because measles is so contagious. Researchers have found that the first MMR dose creates immunity to measles in 95 percent of the people who are vaccinated. The second MMR dose increases immunity to measles to about 99 percent.

> **Brain Booster**
>
> If necessary, your health-care provider can run a blood test to find out whether you have adequate immunity to a disease. Serological testing looks at the levels of antibodies in your blood serum. If you have high levels of antibodies to the disease, you should be protected from infection.

The standard recommended vaccines adults and children might get are about 75 to 99 percent effective at creating immunity to a disease. The level of effectiveness varies with each vaccine. The following information shows how effectively each childhood vaccine creates immunity.

Immunity to Vaccine-Preventable Diseases After Receiving All the Doses of a Childhood Vaccine

Vaccine	% of People Immune to Vaccine Antigens Post-Vaccination (Approximate)
DTaP and Tdap	80% or more to pertussis; 95% to diphtheria; 99% to tetanus
Hepatitis A	94% or more
Hepatitis B	98% or more
Hib	95% or more
HPV	95% to 99%
Influenza (inactivated)	70–90%
Influenza (live)	87% (ages 5 to 7)
Meningococcal (MCV4)	98%
Meningococcal (MPSV4)	67% to over 90%
MMR	99% to measles; 95% to mumps and rubella
Pneumococcal (PCV7)	90% or more
Pneumococcal (PPV23)	60% to 70%
Polio (IPV)	99%
Rotavirus	74% to any rotavirus infection; 98% protected from severe infections
Varicella	70–90% to all chickenpox; 95% against severe chickenpox

Source: The Centers for Disease Control and Prevention, "Parents' Guide to Childhood Immunizations" (updated Feb 2009), and CDC Pink Books.

The best protection against immune response failure is a high vaccination rate in each community. If enough people around you are vaccinated, the herd immunity created by high vaccination levels can make a disease outbreak unlikely. Herd immunity also protects those who cannot receive some vaccinations for medical reasons (such as people with suppressed immune systems), those who have not yet received all the recommended doses of a vaccine (such as young infants), and those who choose not to receive a vaccination for other reasons.

To achieve herd immunity to a disease, vaccination levels in the entire population must be high. It varies with each disease, but in general, about 85 to 95 percent of the population must be immune to a disease to protect those who do not have immunity to a disease.

Tracking Vaccine Safety

As described in Chapter 3, any new vaccines go through a rigorous, multiyear development and testing cycle before they are recommended and available for children or adults. New vaccines are also monitored for problems after they are added to the vaccination schedule because very rare adverse events caused by a vaccine might not show up in the vaccine's clinical trials.

The Vaccine Adverse Events Reporting System (VAERS) was established in 1990 to collect data on illnesses that might be related to vaccines. It enables health-care providers to file a report if certain illnesses, such as shock or brain inflammation, occur after a vaccination. Parents and others can also file a report with the VAERS. This data helps researchers track and analyze any problems that might be caused by either new or established vaccines. Each year in the United States, about 200 million doses of vaccines are given, and the VAERS receives about 20,000 reports of adverse events after vaccination.

VAERS data serves as an "early warning system" that can show whether a vaccine might cause certain adverse events. With data from the VAERS, researchers can look for patterns of certain health problems associated with a vaccine, or investigate claims if the public perceives that certain health problems are related to a vaccine. Researchers can then do further studies to learn whether or not these patterns in the VAERS data indicate a true problem with a vaccine.

Researchers at the Clinical Immunization Safety Assessment (CISA) Center, a network of experts from six research centers in the United States, meet monthly to discuss and respond to serious cases reported to the VAERS. CISA experts also study any possible genetic reasons why a person might become ill from a vaccine.

Vaccinating Facts
Reporting systems such as the VAERS exist in many other countries besides the United States. They provide access to an even larger amount of helpful data about vaccines and side effects. It can be difficult to compare data from different countries, however, because of varying definitions of reportable adverse events. For example, two countries might have different rules for what temperature is high enough to be considered a fever that should be reported. To address this issue, an international organization called the Brighton Collaboration was formed to standardize definitions of adverse events after vaccinations. The Brighton Collaboration is funded by the CDC, the World Health Organization (WHO), and other groups.

The Vaccine Safety Datalink (VSD) project is a key tool that researchers use to look at vaccine safety. The VSD is a linked database of vaccination and other medical information from eight managed care organizations around the United States. The CDC works with the managed care organizations to maintain this database and look for patterns of medical problems associated with vaccines. The VSD is often used to investigate claims filed with the VAERS. But, unlike the VAERS, the VSD also includes health information about people who did not receive the vaccine. This data can help researchers understand how many vaccinated and unvaccinated people had this adverse event.

As a result of this reporting, some vaccines have been removed from the schedule or modified to make serious side effects less likely. For example, an earlier version of the rotavirus vaccine was discontinued after it was linked with a rare intestinal problem, and the pertussis (whooping cough) vaccine was modified to decrease the likelihood that it would cause persistent crying or seizures after vaccination.

Understanding VAERS Data

You can file a report with the VAERS even if you don't know whether the vaccine caused the health problem. Data reported to the VAERS is analyzed by the CDC and a branch of the FDA called the Center for Biologics Evaluation and Research (CBER) to see whether there are any problems consistently linked to certain vaccines.

Brain Booster

The VAERS's information is available to the public. You can search the VAERS data at http://vaers.hhs.gov. You can also file a VAERS report online, or submit a VAERS form by fax at 1-877-721-0366 or by mail at VAERS, PO Box 1100, Rockville, MD, 20849-1100. If you have questions about the VAERS, call the VAERS at 1-800-822-7967 or e-mail info@vaers.org.

Not all the health problems listed in the VAERS are caused by a vaccine. A health problem that occurs after a vaccination might be caused by the vaccine, or it might have happened even if the person wasn't vaccinated. Furthermore, most of the VAERS data is not verified by CDC and CBER officials before it is posted online. VAERS is a passive data collection system, which means that reporting an adverse event after a vaccination is optional in most cases. About 15 percent of the VAERS reports involve serious health problems, such as an illness that requires hospitalization or a severe allergic reaction. The officials investigate these serious problems, but they might not investigate less serious problems such as fevers or headaches.

CDC and CBER officials use the VAERS data to look for patterns of health problems associated with a vaccine. If they see something unusual, they start a formal investigation using more rigorous scientific methods and tools. They gather more information about the relevant VAERS reports and search other databases, such as the VSD, for more information.

VAERS and Vaccine Lots

Vaccine manufacturers create vaccines in batches, or lots, of different sizes. A larger vaccine lot might receive more VAERS reports than a smaller vaccine lot simply because it is larger. Sometimes a number of health problems reported to the VAERS are associated with certain vaccine lots, which is helpful information for investigators.

The FDA licenses and inspects vaccine production facilities, and vaccine manufacturers regularly test their vaccines for safety. When a problem is discovered with a vaccine lot, the FDA stops the distribution and use of vaccines in that lot. These measures help ensure the safety of the vaccines that you receive.

The vaccines used today are extremely safe. They provide protection from life-threatening diseases that might be circulating in your community or that are just a plane ride away in our globally connected world. Today's vaccines have also undergone many years of testing and analysis to ensure that they are as safe as possible.

Some people, however, simply mistrust the pharmaceutical companies that make vaccines, or mistrust the federal agencies charged with recommending and monitoring vaccines. Learning more about how vaccines are developed, tested, and recommended (information covered in Chapter 3) can help put these concerns into perspective.

Getting Help

In the 1970s, there were many lawsuits against the manufacturers of the diphtheria, tetanus, and pertussis (DTP) vaccine because the vaccine caused a range of side effects in children. The vaccine was later reformulated into the diphtheria, tetanus, and acellular pertussis (DTaP) vaccine to alleviate its side effects, and this is the version used today. The lawsuits against the old DTP vaccine created a big problem. Although the old DTP vaccine did cause some serious adverse events, some of the lawsuits were settled without any evidence that the vaccines had indeed caused harm. Because of these costly lawsuits, some vaccine manufacturers stopped making the DTP vaccine. As a result, the price of vaccines increased, causing a shortage of DTP vaccines. In response, in 1984, the CDC recommended postponing the fourth and fifth DTP doses for young children. Although more DTP vaccines became available in 1985, some children did not complete the DTP series of doses and were not fully immunized. If vaccination rates dropped too low due to a shortage caused by a situation like this, the United States would become vulnerable to disease outbreaks.

In response to these problems, the federal government passed the National Childhood Vaccine Injury Act (NCVIA) in 1986. The NCVIA was designed to more easily resolve vaccine-related lawsuits and to support national immunization campaigns (and prevent vaccine shortages) by directing lawsuits away from vaccine manufacturers.

The NCVIA requires that health-care providers give a Vaccine Information Statement to everyone who receives a recommended childhood vaccine (or to their parent or guardian). The statement explains the risks and benefits of the vaccine, including possible side effects. The NCVIA led to the establishment of the VAERS for health-care providers and others to report certain adverse events if they happened after a vaccination. The NCVIA also created a National Vaccine Program Office to coordinate the activities of the different federal agencies that work with vaccines, and created a committee to review existing data on vaccination side effects.

> **Brain Booster**
>
> An adult who receives a vaccine recommended for children, such as the DTaP or MMR vaccine, is also covered under the National Childhood Vaccine Injury Act. If the adult is injured by the vaccine, he or she can seek compensation through the National Vaccine Injury Compensation Program.

Furthermore, the NCVIA set up a National Vaccine Injury Compensation Program (VICP) that would fairly compensate anyone who was injured by a childhood vaccine. The VICP covers injuries from childhood vaccines for 15 diseases: diphtheria, tetanus, pertussis, measles, mumps, rubella, polio, hepatitis B, Hib, varicella (chickenpox), rotavirus, HPV, hepatitis A, meningococcal disease, and pneumococcal disease. The program also covers injuries resulting from influenza vaccines given to both children and adults.

How does the VICP define a vaccine injury? Researchers created a Vaccine Injury Table, based on an extensive review of medical studies of adverse events that occurred after vaccinations. They concluded that certain adverse events that occurred within a certain time frame after a vaccination were probably caused by the vaccination. When someone's vaccine-related injury is listed on the Vaccine Injury Table, and the injury occurred within the time span listed on the table, they can file a claim to be compensated for the cost of the injury, treatment, pain, and suffering, and other expenses.

Some of the injuries listed on the Vaccine Injury Table include:

◆ Life-threatening allergic reactions after DTaP, Tdap, MMR, polio, or hepatitis B vaccinations

◆ Brachial neuritis (severe shoulder pain) after DTaP or Tdap vaccinations

◆ Brain disease or inflammation after DTaP, Tdap, or MMR vaccinations

◆ Chronic arthritis after the MMR vaccination (from the rubella component)

◆ Polio after the OPV (live polio) vaccination

Filing a Claim

The VICP is run by three federal departments: the Department of Health and Human Services, the Department of Justice, and the Court of Federal Claims. All vaccine injury claims are heard by a special master, an authority appointed by a judge to fairly oversee the cases. This "vaccine court" tries to resolve cases quickly to avoid expensive and time-consuming litigation.

If an injury is listed on the Vaccine Injury Table and occurred within the time span listed on the table, a "no fault" claim can be filed, which means a person doesn't need to prove that the vaccine manufacturer or health-care provider is at fault. Instead, the vaccine court assumes that the vaccine might have caused the illness. If nothing else might have caused the illness, such as other medications being taken at the time, compensation can be received for the injuries.

Claims can also be filed for injuries not listed in the table, or when a vaccine on the table worsened another existing medical condition. These claims are more difficult to win because, unlike injuries listed on the table, a person must prove that there is a link between the vaccine and their injury by using scientific studies and other resources. Even if the claim is not compensated, however, it is possible to receive compensation for the legal fees. Claims turned down for compensation can also be appealed through the federal court system.

Brain Booster

The Vaccine Injury Table, and more information about the VICP, is available online at www.hrsa.gov/vaccinecompensation. You can also call 1-800-338-2382 for more information.

Reports of adverse events filed with the VAERS are not automatically entered into the VICP. To be compensated for an injury, a person must file a VICP claim. Historically, the DTP vaccine (which is no longer used in the United States), the MMR vaccine, and the hepatitis B vaccine have had the most claims filed against them.

Over the past few years, the VICP has paid out close to $100 million in claims each year. Where does this money come from? The VICP is funded by a small excise tax charged on every vaccine dose.

Recent Cases

Because recent studies show no link between autism and vaccination, autism and autism spectrum disorders are not listed on the Vaccine Injury Table. Since 2001, however, the VICP has received over 5,500 claims that a vaccine caused autism in a child. Rather than try all these cases separately, the special masters divided these claims into three groups of test cases representing three points of view on autism and vaccines:

◆ The MMR vaccine causes autism when combined with other vaccines containing thimerosal (the MMR vaccine has never contained thimerosal)

◆ The preservative thimerosal causes autism

◆ The MMR vaccine alone causes autism

In early 2009, the special masters released their conclusion on whether MMR and thimerosal together can cause autism. They concluded that MMR and thimerosal did not cause autism.

In 2008, a different VICP case also raised questions about vaccines and autism. A girl named Hannah Poling had received five vaccinations at once, including the MMR vaccination, when she was about one and a half years old. After the vaccinations, she became ill and feverish, and several months later she developed autism-like symptoms. It was discovered that the root cause of her symptoms, however, was encephalopathy (brain disease) caused by mitochondrial disease, an illness in which the body does not produce enough energy for all its cells.

Because the brain uses a lot of energy, mitochondrial disease often causes neurological symptoms. The disease can be triggered by problems such as infections or stress. The special masters decided that the vaccinations might have triggered or aggravated Poling's mitochondrial disease; therefore, the Poling family received compensation for Hannah's injury. You can learn more about the Hannah Poling case in the article "Vaccines and Autism Revisited—The Hannah Poling Case," written by Dr. Paul Offit and published in *The New England Journal of Medicine* in 2008. It is available online at http://content.nejm.org/cgi/content/full/358/20/2089.

The Least You Need to Know

♦ In rare instances, vaccines can cause serious or life-threatening illnesses.

♦ Some people who get vaccinated will not develop immunity to a disease.

♦ The federal government collects and analyzes data on illnesses related to vaccines.

♦ A special vaccine court exists to compensate those injured by certain vaccines.

Chapter 15

Funding Vaccines

In This Chapter

- ◆ Why vaccine research and manufacturing is under-funded
- ◆ How funding shortages create vaccine shortages
- ◆ How federal and state governments are working to solve funding issues
- ◆ How developing countries handle vaccine funding issues

Vaccines benefit public health, and they are created in the business sector by just a few private manufacturers. Therefore, they must be profitable in order for manufacturers to keep making them. Vaccines also must be widely available and used to effectively control infectious diseases and improve public health. To ensure widespread vaccination for the public good, federal and state governments negotiate vaccine prices and subsidize many childhood vaccines for families who can't afford them.

Lower prices, fears of litigation, and other factors have reduced the competition to create vaccines, discouraged new research, and made the vaccine program vulnerable to shortages. New funding strategies used by developing countries, such as guaranteed vaccine purchase, have encouraged vaccine manufacturers to continue to work on them for the public good. To make the national vaccination program more robust in the United States, however, the public needs to agree to pay more for the value that vaccines provide to society.

Research and Manufacturing

Vaccines are not just extremely successful at preventing disease; they are also a good public health investment. According to a 2005 study in the *Archives of Pediatrics & Adolescent Medicine*, for every dollar spent on childhood vaccines in the United States, about $17 are saved on the health-care and societal costs of treating a vaccine-preventable disease and its consequences.

For vaccine manufacturers, however, vaccine development is not very profitable. The pharmaceutical companies that develop and manufacture them make more money from other drugs, such as medications that lower cholesterol or treat heartburn. A pharmaceutical company's "blockbuster" drug can earn over $1 billion each year—far more than any vaccine can earn. Lawsuits filed over vaccines such as the old diphtheria, tetanus, and pertussis (DTP) vaccine drove some vaccine manufacturers to stop making vaccines altogether for fear of litigation. In the 1970s, 25 pharmaceutical companies made the vaccines sold in the United States; by the end of 2008, there were only 6.

> **Brain Booster**
>
> There are over 100 "blockbuster" drugs on the market today, earning pharmaceutical manufacturers more than $100 billion each year.

Having fewer vaccine manufacturers creates a number of problems. First of all, it makes for limited competition to create vaccines. For some vaccines, such as the measles, mumps, and rubella (MMR) vaccine, there is only one U.S. manufacturer. If a manufacturer has problems making a vaccine, there can be vaccine shortages because few or no other manufacturers can step in to supplement the supply. Also, legal and regulatory issues can make it difficult to import needed vaccines made in other countries.

Second, the United States government purchases vaccines in bulk to distribute in several federal vaccination programs. Because the government buys in bulk, it negotiates discounts that make vaccines less profitable for manufacturers. Tightened Food and Drug Administration (FDA) rules regarding how vaccines are made and approved also make it more expensive to create a vaccine now than in the past. As a result, vaccine manufacturers have limited financial motivations to create new vaccines or improve older ones.

Collaboration between vaccine manufacturers and the government has helped solve some of these problems. For example, the National Childhood Vaccine Injury Act (NCVIA) of 1986, discussed in Chapter 14, was designed to provide compensation for children injured by vaccines, while protecting manufacturers from damaging lawsuits, and to ensure that manufacturers would continue to make vaccines. The NCVIA has been effective in protecting both the national vaccination program and children injured by vaccines.

Federal programs designed to pay for more children to get vaccines help ensure that there will be a market for all recommended childhood vaccines. Vaccine manufacturers also draw on publicly funded vaccine research to improve vaccines and continue developing new ones.

Distribution

The more people who are vaccinated against a disease, the greater the benefit for public health. It can be difficult, however, to provide vaccines for everyone who should get one. Many vaccines have been added to the schedule of recommended childhood vaccines within the past 20 years. Scientific advances have made this possible. But these advances, along with increased safety regulations (such as larger clinical trials), have made new vaccines more expensive to produce than older vaccines.

In 1985, it cost the federal government $45 to buy all the childhood vaccines that one child needed from newborn to age 18 (according to the vaccination funding advocacy group The 317 Coalition). Because the number and price of childhood vaccines has increased since then, it is now much more expensive for the government to purchase these vaccines. In 2007, according to The 317 Coalition, the federal government needed to pay $924 for the childhood vaccines for a boy, and $1,214 for the childhood vaccines for a girl (girls include the three-dose human papillomavirus vaccine).

Private Health Plans

Vaccines can be expensive for health-care providers within private health-care plans as well. Sometimes, the plans do not reimburse the providers at a high enough rate to cover the cost of purchasing and administering the vaccine. Vaccination coverage for individuals varies by health plan, and some plans do not cover the cost of adult or childhood vaccinations, making patients pay out of pocket for this expense. The federal government is considering removing barriers to childhood vaccination for people with private health insurance. The Comprehensive Insurance Coverage of Childhood Immunization Act of 2009 (H.R. 323) is an attempt to make vaccines more affordable and accessible for people with group or individual health insurance. This bill builds on recommendations from a 2003 report from the Institute of Medicine, *Financing Vaccines in the 21st Century*, and would require that private insurers cover the cost of all recommended childhood vaccinations. Some states currently have this requirement, while others do not; a federal law, as a result of this bill, would apply to all the states. Under the bill, the vaccinations must be fully covered, and the private insurers could not charge patients co-pays or co-insurance. If the bill is passed, it would take effect on January 1, 2010.

Government Health Plans

From 1989 to 1991, a measles outbreak swept through the United States, infecting over 55,000 people and causing 123 deaths. The outbreak especially impacted children in minority and urban communities. About half of the people who caught measles were under five years old, an age group that had low measles vaccination rates at the time. Ninety percent of the people who died from measles during this outbreak were not vaccinated against the disease.

This outbreak triggered an increased effort to vaccinate young children against measles in the United States. The federal government stepped in, and legislation was passed to provide free vaccines to underinsured children. Today, half of the childhood vaccines used in the United States are bought by the federal government and are distributed to the individual states through several vaccination programs.

The Vaccines for Children (VFC) program, enacted in 1994, provides free vaccines to certain groups of children:

- Children on Medicaid, the health insurance program for low-income families that is funded by both federal and state governments

- Children who are uninsured

- Children of Alaskan Native or American Indian heritage

Underinsured children can also get free vaccines through the VFC program if there is a federally funded health clinic in their area. Although the vaccines are free, families might need to pay a small administrative fee for each vaccine.

People who do not qualify for the VFC program might be able to get free childhood vaccinations through Section 317 of the Public Health Services Act. Section 317 gives grants to individual states to help them purchase vaccines and run vaccine-related programs, such as public outreach campaigns. Section 317 funds help states purchase childhood vaccines and some adult vaccines for people who cannot afford them.

Brain Booster

To join the Vaccines for Children (VFC) program in your area, contact your state or territory VFC coordinator. Go to www.cdc. gov/vaccines/programs/ vfc/contacts-state.htm or call the CDC at 1-800-232-4636 to find your VFC coordinator. This person can answer questions and enroll you in the VFC program.

Some states provide free vaccines only for people whose health insurance does not cover vaccinations, or for people who don't have insurance. Other states follow a universal purchase program, providing free childhood vaccines to all the children in the state (like the VFC program, the vaccines are free, but patients pay an administrative fee).

Unfortunately, federal Section 317 funding has not kept pace with the increasing cost of vaccines. Before 2000, it covered the cost of childhood vaccines for those who could not afford them and those who didn't qualify for the VFC program. Since then, however, as more vaccines were added to the childhood vaccination schedule and vaccine costs rose, federal Section 317 funding has not kept up with these costs. To continue their vaccination programs, states must contribute more money from their own budgets, which may or may not be happening. Therefore, some families that can't afford to vaccinate their children are not covered, and their children remain unvaccinated.

Vaccinating Facts
Every 10 years, the U.S. Department of Health and Human Services (HHS) creates health goals for the nation as part of its Healthy People program. The Healthy People 2010 goals include eliminating most vaccine-preventable childhood diseases, and greatly decreasing the number of cases of hepatitis B, pertussis, and varicella (chickenpox) in children.

Developing Countries

Funding vaccines in developing countries is especially difficult because they have such limited public health budgets to pay for them. Because they won't make much profit from them, vaccine manufacturers can be unwilling to develop vaccines that are needed in the developing world, such as a malaria vaccine, that are not needed in wealthier countries.

To supply vaccines to the developing world, vaccine manufacturers charge different prices for them than in wealthier countries. Although they might lose money on the vaccines they sell in developing countries, this is offset by profits they get from wealthier countries. To provide vaccines for developing countries, international organizations such as the United Nations Children's Fund (UNICEF) negotiate lower prices for large vaccine purchases from the manufacturers.

These vaccine pricing practices, however, make it less likely that a manufacturer will develop a vaccine (such as the malaria vaccine) that is not needed in wealthier countries. If the manufacturer can't subsidize low costs by selling the vaccine in a wealthier country as well, it can be hard for them to recover the cost of developing the vaccine. Furthermore, the developing world still uses some types of vaccines, such as the old diphtheria, tetanus, and pertussis (DTP) vaccine, that are no longer used in wealthier countries. Newer vaccines are more expensive for developing countries to purchase than older vaccines. As a result, it can be hard for developing countries to:

◆ Get access to older vaccines no longer used in wealthier countries.

◆ Get access to existing newer vaccines.

◆ Persuade manufacturers to develop new vaccines for diseases that are rare in wealthier countries.

Distributing vaccines can also be difficult in some developing countries. Effective distribution depends on an adequate health-care infrastructure. Widespread vaccination against a disease requires both government coordination and the cooperation of local communities. Countries with weak or overburdened governments may find it difficult to conduct a vaccination campaign. Vaccine-preventable diseases sometimes break out in countries engaged in a civil war, for example, because war displaces people and disrupts transportation, communication, and health-care services.

Vaccinating Facts

In an effort to eliminate polio worldwide, many developing countries promote National Immunization Days. In 2005, for example, over 15 million young children in Ethiopia were vaccinated against polio during several National Immunization Days, according to the World Health Organization. Some countries in the middle of civil wars, such as El Salvador, Sri Lanka, and Angola, have declared cease-fires to ensure that these vaccinations take place.

Furthermore, sometimes community members must be educated about the benefits of a vaccine before they agree to be vaccinated. There must be adequate health-care providers in each community to administer the vaccine as well, which can be a challenge if people live in remote locations or have a nomadic lifestyle.

To overcome these problems, philanthropic organizations such as the Bill & Melinda Gates Foundation raise money to pay for the development of new vaccines (for malaria, tuberculosis, HIV/AIDS, and other diseases) needed in the developing world. Other organizations, such as the Global Alliance for Vaccines and Immunization (GAVI), coordinate public-private partnerships that include private organizations, government agencies, and vaccine manufacturers to bring vaccines to developing countries.

Certain financial incentives can also help bring needed vaccines to developing countries. GAVI supports a practice called Advance Market Commitment, in which they promise to purchase a certain number of doses of a new vaccine that developing countries need at a fair (not reduced) price. This encourages manufacturers to create these vaccines because they know they will make a profit from them. To encourage investment in vaccination programs for developing countries, some countries, such as the United Kingdom, are financing "vaccine bonds." With these bonds, countries pledge money to support vaccination programs in developing countries for 10 to 20 years, and then issue bonds against this pledge.

Vaccine Shortages

Vaccine shortages can happen for a number of reasons. Most often it's because a manufacturer is unable to produce vaccines due to a problem or contamination in a manufacturing facility. The vaccine production might be stopped and the vaccines recalled for safety reasons. If no other vaccines (such as a combination vaccine) can replace this supply, there can be a shortage of the vaccine.

Vaccine shortages can be confusing and frustrating for patients and their families. Shortages also place an extra burden on health-care providers. Fortunately, though, vaccine shortages in the United States have not yet caused any outbreaks of vaccine-preventable diseases.

New safety or production regulations can also slow down the manufacturing process, causing a delay in vaccine availability. Or, the demand for a vaccine might be higher than anticipated one year, and the manufacturer might not be able to meet this demand. If a new vaccine is added to the childhood vaccination schedule, for example, manufacturers might not be able to keep up with the initial demand. Problems as diverse as a natural disaster or corporate restructuring within a vaccine manufacturing company can lead to vaccine shortages.

In theory, a problem with one vaccine manufacturer would not have a large impact on the supply of vaccines in the United States if there were many other manufacturers who were also producing the vaccine. For example, if 10 manufacturers each supplied 10 percent of the Hib vaccines, then a problem with 1 manufacturer would only affect 10 percent of the Hib vaccine supply. Today, however, there are only two Hib manufacturers.

Vaccine shortages do happen periodically in the United States. From 2000 to 2003, for example, there were shortages of vaccines for eight childhood diseases.

Recent Shortages

The Hib vaccine made by Merck was recalled in 2007 after Merck found bacteria on some of its vaccine manufacturing equipment. Because Merck supplied half of the Hib vaccines used in the United States, this recall created a shortage of the Hib vaccine. This shortage continued into 2009; as a result, there were not enough Hib doses to follow the childhood vaccination recommendations for all children.

In response, the CDC created interim recommendations for the Hib vaccine. The agency recommended deferring the last Hib dose for healthy children, given when a child is 12 to 15 months old, in order to conserve the vaccine. Children at higher risk of developing a Hib infection, such as those with leukemia or HIV infections, did receive the last Hib dose to give them the highest level of immunity to Hib infection.

Brain Booster

The latest vaccine shortages and delays are posted on the CDC website at www.cdc.gov/vaccines/vac-gen/shortages/default.htm.

The CDC often responds to vaccine shortages by temporarily reducing the number of recommended doses. This saves doses for children and adults at highest risk of catching a vaccine-preventable disease and makes more of the vaccine available overall.

During a well-publicized shortage of the influenza vaccine from 2004 to 2005, the English influenza vaccine manufacturer Chiron had manufacturing problems, cutting that year's influenza vaccine supply in half in the United States. The Advisory Committee on Immunization Practices (ACIP) recommended prioritizing influenza vaccination during that influenza season for people at highest risk of being seriously harmed by influenza, such as certain health-care workers who could accidentally give the flu to their patients, and people who lived or worked with children under six months old. This move protected the people most vulnerable to influenza complications.

Brain Booster

To find out whether there is a shortage of a travel vaccine, visit the CDC's Travelers' Health website at wwwn.cdc.gov/travel/.

Vaccine shortages don't just occur among vaccines for children. There can be shortages of vaccines for other groups as well, including travelers' vaccines, such as the yellow fever vaccine. A 2008 to 2009 shortage of the rabies vaccine, for example, limited the amount of pre-exposure (prophylactic) vaccines available.

The Vaccine Stockpile

In 1983, the federal government began a national vaccine stockpile program as part of the Vaccines for Children program. The program was designed to contain enough doses of vaccines to supply all the recommended childhood vaccines for all United States children for six months. The government contracts with vaccine manufacturers, who maintain fresh doses of childhood vaccines for the stockpile. If there were a vaccine shortage, the government could distribute the vaccines as needed.

The government has used the stockpile numerous times to respond to vaccine shortages or to increase vaccination rates during outbreaks of vaccine-preventable diseases. In 2009, for example, the CDC released doses of hepatitis B vaccine from the stockpile when the demand for the vaccine exceeded the manufacturer's supplies.

Today, the stockpile does not contain six months' worth of vaccines for every vaccine on the recommended childhood vaccination schedule.

Funding problems, administrative issues, and changes to the child-hood vaccination schedule have made it difficult to maintain the stock-pile. Instead, the stockpile just contains supplies of the vaccines most vulnerable to shortages. The stockpile contains adequate doses of the MMR vaccine, for example, because it is only made by Merck and no other vaccine manufacturers could provide the vaccine if Merck had a manufacturing problem. The stockpile contains some doses (but not six months' worth) of many other vaccines, such as DTaP.

Future Funding Strategies

As federal and state budgets shrink in the United States, the number and cost of recommended childhood vaccines have risen. As a result, there are funding gaps for vaccine programs and for the vaccine stock-pile. Liability concerns and market forces limit the amount of invest-ment vaccine manufacturers make in developing new vaccines and improving existing ones.

Because vaccination programs prevent disease outbreaks, their successes are often invisible to the public, especially since life-threatening infec-tious diseases are quite rare now in the United States. When the first polio vaccination campaign began in the 1950s, everyone knew some-one who had had polio, and many people saw first-hand its devastating impact. Today, however, most adults in the United States don't know anyone who has caught polio, measles, diphtheria, or many other vaccine-preventable diseases. Vaccinating a healthy child or adult against a disease they probably wouldn't catch seems illogical to some people.

Now other childhood diseases such as autism and asthma are far more visible than many infectious diseases more prevalent in days past. If current vaccination rates drop, however, many of these infectious dis-eases could come back. The outbreak of measles in 2008, the worst outbreak in years, proves that these diseases could easily return to the United States.

Some public health researchers believe that the public doesn't value vaccines as much as they should. When people don't see the value of vaccines, they don't ask their federal and state governments to make vaccine funding a priority. If the public valued vaccines enough to pay higher prices for them, it could provide more incentives for vaccine manufacturers to invest in new and existing vaccines.

To a degree, solving funding problems with vaccines comes down to showing people that vaccines are a critical public health achievement that has saved—and has continued to save—millions of lives. Vaccine research can benefit from better public education about the value of vaccines. When people understand their value, they are more likely to ask for more generous federal allocations for and investments in vaccine research and distribution.

The Least You Need to Know

♦ Many manufacturers have stopped making vaccines because they are not very profitable for them.

♦ Federal funding policies that support widespread vaccination sometimes undermine vaccine research.

♦ Some philanthropic organizations use financial tools to reward vaccine innovation and distribution in developing countries.

♦ In the United States, vaccines need to be valued publicly in order for manufacturers to keep making and improving vaccines.

Glossary

acquired immunodeficiency syndrome (AIDS) Severe illness caused by immune system damage due to advanced human immunodeficiency virus (HIV) infection.

active infection An infection that causes symptoms and that can be passed on to others.

acute illness An illness that lasts for a short time (from days to months) and usually does not cause long-term problems.

adaptive immune system The part of the immune system with cells that can change to fight different threats. Because certain cells "remember" these threats in case they return, long-term immunity to diseases is created within the adaptive immune system.

adjuvant A vaccine additive that acts as a minor irritant to enhance an immune system's response to the vaccine.

Advance Market Commitment A funding strategy for developing countries in which an organization agrees to purchase a set amount of new vaccines from a vaccine manufacturer at a fair market price.

adverse event An illness or injury that occurs after getting a vaccination or other medical treatments.

Advisory Committee on Immunization Practices (ACIP)   A group of 15 experts appointed by the federal government to update and maintain the vaccination recommendation schedules in the United States.

allergic reaction   A type of systemic (body-wide) reaction to a vaccine or any other foreign substance that can be life-threatening.

anaphylactic shock   A life-threatening condition caused by an allergic reaction. It can cause breathing problems and can be fatal.

anthrax   A potentially fatal bacterial disease that can spread from animals to humans. Anthrax can be spread by contact with infected animal products (cutaneous anthrax), by eating infected meat (gastrointestinal anthrax), or by inhaling anthrax spores (inhalation anthrax).

antibiotics   Medications used to stop bacterial infections.

antibody   A substance created by the adaptive immune system's B cells that reacts to antigens.

antigen   The part of a pathogenic virus, bacterium, or other substance that triggers the immune system to respond. They are called "antigens" because they are *anti*body-*gen*erating substances.

antiretroviral drugs   Medications used to slow the progression of the retrovirus human immunodeficiency virus (HIV) to acquired immunodeficiency syndrome (AIDS).

Asperger's syndrome   A type of autism spectrum disorder that includes socialization and behavioral symptoms.

asthma   A chronic illness that causes airway inflammation. Asthma can cause problems such as coughing and wheezing.

attenuated   Weakened.

autism   A developmental disorder marked by problems with communication, socialization, and behavior.

autism spectrum disorders (ASDs)   A group of developmental disorders that includes autism and Asperger's syndrome.

B cell   A cell in the adaptive immune system that creates antibodies to catch antigens.

Bacille Calmette-Guérin (BCG) vaccine A vaccine that provides limited protection against pulmonary tuberculosis. The BCG vaccine has never been a standard vaccination in the United States.

bacterium A simple, very common organism that can be helpful or harmful (pathogenic) to humans. "Bacteria" is the plural form of the word.

BCG vaccine *See* Bacille Calmette-Guérin.

brachial neuritis Severe shoulder pain that can be caused by a vaccine on rare occasions.

Center for Biologics Evaluation and Research (CBER) A division of the Food and Drug Administration (FDA) that regulates vaccines.

Centers for Disease Control and Prevention (CDC) A government organization that promotes safety and health in the United States.

chickenpox *See* varicella.

cholera A bacterial disease common in some developing countries that can cause severe diarrhea and other problems. A cholera vaccine is not currently available in the United States.

chronic illness An illness that lasts more than three months or that comes and goes over time.

Clinical Immunization Safety Assessment (CISA) Center Network A group of experts who review and respond to Vaccine Adverse Event Reporting System (VAERS) data on a monthly basis. VAERS collects data on health problems that occur after vaccinations.

clinical trials A series of tests designed to see whether a vaccine or medicine is safe and effective before it is licensed for use. Clinical trials, which follow strict rules for safety and ethics, are done on groups of human volunteers.

combination vaccine A vaccine that provides immunity to several diseases at once, such as the measles, mumps, and rubella (MMR) vaccine.

Commission on Clinical Policies and Research (CCRP) A group of experts from the American Academy of Family Physicians who make recommendations regarding vaccine policy.

Committee on Infectious Diseases (COID) A group of experts from the American Academy of Pediatrics who make recommendations regarding vaccine policy.

Comprehensive Insurance Coverage of Childhood Immunization Act of 2009 (H.R. 323) Proposed legislation that would require that private health-care insurers cover the cost of vaccinations.

congenital rubella syndrome (CRS) A group of birth defects, such as deafness and mental retardation, that can occur in a newborn if the mother is infected with the rubella virus when she is pregnant.

conjugate vaccine A vaccine that combines antigens with a biological carrier to make it more effective; especially useful for young children, who do not respond to polysaccharide vaccines until two years of age.

contact immunity Gaining immunity to a disease by being in close contact with someone who received a live vaccine.

Cutter Laboratories A vaccine manufacturer in Berkeley, California, that had a manufacturing problem with the polio vaccine in the 1950s.

diabetes A chronic disease that affects the body's ability to control the level of sugar in the blood.

diphtheria A vaccine-preventable bacterial disease that can cause breathing and swallowing problems. Diphtheria is sometimes fatal.

DNA (deoxyribonucleic acid) vaccine A vaccine that contains the genetic code for an antigen. Human cells use the code to make the antigen and trigger an immune response. DNA vaccines are currently experimental only.

edible vaccines Vaccines incorporated into genetically modified foods, such as bananas. Edible vaccines are still in development, but they would be simpler and cheaper to produce than injected vaccines.

encephalitis An inflammation of the brain, usually caused by a virus or bacteria. Symptoms of encephalitis can include fever, a stiff neck, headache, confusion, vomiting, and sensitivity to light.

epidemic A regional increase in the number of cases of an infectious disease.

extensively drug-resistant tuberculosis (XDR TB) A type of tuberculosis that does not respond to any antibiotics.

extrapulmonary tuberculosis Tuberculosis that affects the brain, kidneys, and other body parts.

Food and Drug Administration (FDA) A federal organization that licenses and monitors vaccines, among other functions.

fungi A group of plantlike organisms—including mold, mildew, mushrooms, and yeast—that are sometimes harmful to humans. There are no vaccines against fungi.

Global Alliance for Vaccines and Immunization (GAVI) An organization that coordinates efforts to bring needed vaccines to developing countries.

Guillain-Barré Syndrome (GBS) A rare neurological problem that can cause temporary paralysis. In extremely rare instances, GBS can be fatal.

***Haemophilus influenzae* type b (Hib)** A vaccine-preventable bacterial infection that can cause serious brain and lung infections in children.

hepatitis Liver inflammation. Hepatitis can be caused by alcohol consumption, viral infections, or other problems.

hepatitis A Liver inflammation caused by the hepatitis A virus. Hepatitis A can cause acute (short-term) and severe health problems. Vaccination can prevent hepatitis A infection.

hepatitis B Liver inflammation caused by the hepatitis B virus. Chronic hepatitis B can cause liver cancer. Vaccination can prevent hepatitis B infection.

hepatitis C Liver inflammation caused by the hepatitis C virus, which can lead to liver damage. There is no vaccine for hepatitis C.

herd immunity Group immunity to a disease, created by high vaccination rates within a population. Herd immunity is sometimes called community immunity.

human diploid cells Human cells taken from aborted fetuses and modified to help create some vaccines.

human immunodeficiency virus (HIV) A virus, usually spread by sexual contact, that attacks the immune system. If untreated, HIV leads to acquired immunodeficiency syndrome (AIDS) and other secondary infections.

human papillomavirus (HPV) A group of sexually transmitted viruses, some of which can cause cancer or genital warts. The HPV vaccine protects against four of these types of viruses that are most likely to cause disease.

hypothesis A theory that a scientist tries to prove or disprove through experiments and data analysis.

immune globulin A blood product containing antibodies to a disease. Immune globulin can provide short-term protection from a disease.

immune system The system of cells and organs that protects the body from pathogens. The immune system includes physical defenses such as skin, specialized cells that capture and destroy dangerous substances, and organs that create and store these specialized cells.

immunity Resistance to an infectious disease.

immunization Vaccination.

inactivated vaccine A vaccine made with killed (inactivated) antigens from viruses or bacteria. Inactivated vaccines often require booster shots to maintain immunity.

incubate To grow and replicate within the body.

incubation period The period of time when a virus or bacteria reproduces in your body but does not yet cause symptoms. Vaccination during an incubation period can sometimes stop or diminish the effects of a disease.

influenza A viral disease that usually causes moderate respiratory symptoms that last for about a week. In certain people, especially children and the elderly, influenza can cause serious complications and death.

innate immune system A part of your immune system that includes cells that can destroy some pathogens.

inoculation   Using a small amount of biological material to trigger an immune response and create immunity to a disease.

Institute of Medicine   A nonprofit organization that advises the federal government on medicine, health, and medical science.

Intensified Global Eradication Program (IGEP)   A program created by the World Health Assembly to eliminate smallpox worldwide. The IGEP achieved this goal by 1980.

International Certificate of Vaccination or Prophylaxis (ICVP)
A document that proves you have received the yellow fever vaccination.

intussusception   A rare bowel problem in children that was linked to an early (now discontinued) rotavirus vaccine.

Japanese encephalitis   A vaccine-preventable viral disease that occurs in South and Southeast Asia and is spread by mosquitoes. Japanese encephalitis can cause brain inflammation and brain damage, and it can be fatal.

jaundice   Yellowing of the skin or eyes caused by liver problems.

Kawasaki disease   A rare childhood disease that causes inflamed arteries and that can cause serious problems such as heart disease.

latent infection   An infection that does not cause symptoms and that cannot be transmitted to someone else.

live vaccine   A vaccine that contains live but weakened (attenuated) antigens from viruses or bacteria. Live vaccines create long-term immunity.

local reaction   A physical response—such as redness, pain, or swelling—at the vaccine injection site.

lymphocytes   A group of adaptive immune system cells that include B cells and T cells.

malaria   An infectious disease spread by mosquitoes that can cause fever, fatigue, and muscle aches. Malaria can be fatal. Malaria is common in many parts of the world. Currently, there is no licensed malaria vaccine, but medications can help travelers avoid infection.

measles   A very contagious vaccine-preventable viral disease that causes a rash and that can lead to serious, sometimes fatal complications.

Medicaid   A federal health-care program for low-income families.

memory cell   An immune system cell that remains in the blood after an antigen is destroyed. Memory cells can quickly stop any future infections with that antigen.

meningitis   An infection of the lining of the brain and spinal cord, usually caused by a virus or bacteria. Symptoms of meningitis can include a stiff neck, high fever, headache, vomiting, confusion, and sensitivity to light.

meningococcal vaccine   A vaccine that prevents infections caused by the *Neisseria meningitidis* bacteria. The newer meningococcal conjugate vaccine (MCV4) is believed to be more effective and offers longer-lasting protection than the meningococcal polysaccharide vaccine (MPSV4).

multidrug-resistant tuberculosis (MDR TB)   A type of tuberculosis that is difficult to treat with commonly used tuberculosis antibiotics.

multiple sclerosis (MS)   A neurological disorder that causes symptoms such as trouble walking and numbness.

mumps   A vaccine-preventable viral disease that causes swollen neck glands and that can lead to serious complications.

mutation   When a cell changes its genetic information, often causing a change in how it replicates.

National Childhood Vaccine Injury Act (NCVIA)   A federal law designed to support the national immunization program in the United States and to provide for people injured by vaccines.

National Vaccine Injury Compensation Program (NVICP or VICP)   A program created by the National Childhood Vaccine Injury Act (NCVIA) to compensate people for legitimate vaccine-related injuries caused by childhood vaccines.

Neisseria meningitidis   A bacterium that can cause rapid, sometimes-fatal infections, such as meningitis. The meningococcal vaccine can prevent infection with this bacterium.

neonatal tetanus   Tetanus infection in newborn babies whose mothers are not vaccinated against tetanus.

organism   A living thing that is one cell or larger. An organism can absorb nutrients and reproduce.

pandemic   A worldwide outbreak of an infectious disease such as influenza.

parasite   An organism that lives on or in another organism during part of its life cycle.

pathogen   A substance that can cause illness in humans or animals.

pertussis   A sometimes-fatal, vaccine-preventable bacterial infection that can cause breathing problems. Pertussis is also called whooping cough.

phagocyte   A type of immune system cell that can destroy bacteria and other cells by ingesting them.

placebo   A harmless substance given to someone in place of a vaccine or medication, usually during clinical trials. Placebos are needed to test the safety and effectiveness of vaccines and medications by comparing people who received the product to those who did not.

pneumococcal bacteria   Bacteria that can cause serious problems such as pneumonia or meningitis. The pneumococcal conjugate vaccine provides protection against these bacteria for children, and the pneumococcal polysaccharide vaccine provides protection for adults.

pneumonia   A lung infection, usually caused by viruses or bacteria.

polio (poliomyelitis)   A vaccine-preventable viral disease that can cause paralysis; can be fatal.

polysaccharide vaccine   A vaccine, such as the pneumococcal polysaccharide vaccine (PPV), containing antigens that are sugars on the shell of a pathogen.

prophylactic   Preventative.

prophylactic vaccine   A vaccine designed to create protective immunity to an infectious disease before an individual is exposed to it. All vaccines on the immunization schedule are prophylactic vaccines.

pulmonary tuberculosis Tuberculosis that affects the lungs.

rabid Infected with the rabies virus.

rabies A fatal virus that can be transmitted from infected animals to humans. Vaccination before or after exposure to rabies can prevent the disease.

recombinant vaccine A DNA or subunit vaccine that uses a biological vector such as a virus to deliver the vaccine to the cells.

replication When an organism makes a copy of itself to reproduce.

rotavirus A virus that can cause vomiting, diarrhea, and dehydration in young children.

rubella A vaccine-preventable viral disease that can cause birth defects and other problems if a pregnant woman becomes infected.

Section 317 of the Public Health Services Act A federal fund that gives grants to states that they can spend on their vaccination programs.

sepsis Infection of the blood.

shingles Rash and nerve pain caused by reactivation of a previous chickenpox infection. Shingles is more common in older adults. The zoster vaccine can prevent shingles.

smallpox A viral infectious disease that is fatal about 30 percent of the time. The first smallpox vaccine was created in the 1790s. Smallpox has now been eradicated worldwide.

spleen An organ that creates some immune system cells and filters your blood.

Study to Explore Early Development (SEED) An ongoing, nationwide, five-year study of developmental disorders, run by the Centers for Disease Control and Prevention (CDC).

subunit vaccine A vaccine that uses part of a virus or a bacterium (rather than the whole pathogen) to trigger an immune response.

Sudden Infant Death Syndrome (SIDS) Sudden death with no clear cause, in an infant under one year old.

systemic reaction A reaction to a vaccine in areas beyond the injection site. Signs of a systemic reaction might include fever, nausea, or headache.

T cell A lymphocyte (a cell in the adaptive immune system) that can destroy cells with certain antigens.

tetanus A vaccine-preventable bacterial disease that can cause fatal breathing problems.

therapeutic vaccine A vaccine given after a disease is diagnosed that is designed to slow or stop the progression of the disease. Therapeutic vaccines are only experimental at this point.

thimerosal A vaccine preservative that contains mercury. Thimerosal was taken out of most vaccines by 2001.

toxin (bacterial) A substance created by bacteria that can be harmful to humans.

toxoid vaccine A vaccine that uses an inactivated (killed) bacterial toxin to create immunity.

tuberculosis A bacterial infection that can affect the lungs or other parts of the body. The current vaccine for tuberculosis has limited effectiveness.

typhoid fever A vaccine-preventable bacterial disease that causes a high fever and other health problems. Typhoid fever is common in some parts of the developing world.

vaccination An inoculation used to create protection against disease. Initially, vaccination referred to smallpox inoculation, but it now refers to all inoculations.

vaccine A biological substance that creates immunity to a viral or bacterial disease. Modern vaccines contain antigens as well as other ingredients such as preservatives and stabilizers.

Vaccine Adverse Event Reporting System (VAERS) A passive data collection system used to monitor health problems that occur after vaccinations.

vaccine bonds Bonds issued against a country's pledge to finance vaccination programs in a developing country for a set amount of time.

Vaccine Injury Table   A list of injuries related to childhood vaccines that are eligible for compensation under the National Vaccine Injury Compensation Program.

Vaccine Safety Datalink (VSD)   A database containing patient data from eight managed care organizations that is used to investigate claims of vaccine-related injuries and illnesses.

vaccine stockpile   A federal program designed to stockpile six months' worth of childhood vaccinations in case of a shortage.

Vaccines for Children   A federal program that provides free vaccines to children in need.

vaccinia virus   A virus that can create immunity to smallpox in humans.

varicella, varicella zoster, or **herpes zoster**   The virus that causes chickenpox and shingles. Chickenpox causes an itchy rash and other symptoms, and can cause serious complications. The varicella vaccine protects against chickenpox.

variola virus   The virus that causes smallpox.

variolation   Inoculation against smallpox using the variola (smallpox) virus. Variolation was an early form of vaccination.

vector   An insect or animal that transmits disease to humans, or a piece of biological material used to carry a vaccine to the cells.

virus   A cell-like organism that uses other cells to perform its life functions. Some viruses are harmful to humans, and others are not.

whooping cough   Pertussis, a vaccine-preventable bacterial disease.

yellow fever   A vaccine-preventable viral disease spread by mosquitoes. Yellow fever causes liver inflammation and can be fatal. It is common in some parts of the world.

zoster   *See* shingles.

Further Reading

General Information About Vaccines

Learn more about vaccines at the Centers for Disease Control and Prevention's comprehensive Vaccines & Immunizations web page, at www.cdc.gov/vaccines. You can also call the CDC's National Immunization Hotline for information, at 1-800-CDC-INFO. The TTY (text telephone) number for the hotline is 1-888-232-6348.

The National Network for Immunization Information, an independent organization not funded by vaccine manufacturers or the government, provides detailed information on each vaccine at www.immunizationinfo.org.

Every Child By Two, an organization co-founded by former First Lady Rosalynn Carter, provides information on vaccines and advocates for federal vaccination policies at www.ecbt.org.

"The What to Expect Guide to Immunizations," a booklet on childhood vaccinations published by the nonprofit What to Expect Foundation, is available at www.whattoexpect.org. The booklet is available in English and Spanish.

The Vaccine Education Center at the Children's Hospital of Philadelphia has information on children's vaccines and vaccination issues at www.vaccine.chop.edu.

The Allied Vaccine Group, a collaboration between several vaccination organizations including the American Academy of Pediatrics, provides information about vaccines and vaccine controversies at www.vaccine. org.

The CDC's online slide shows, "The ABCs of Childhood Vaccines," provide information about vaccines for parents. They are available at www.cdc.gov/vaccines/vac-gen/ABCs/default.htm.

Learn more about the anthrax vaccine for the military at the Department of Defense's website for the Anthrax Vaccine Immunization Program (AVIP) at www.anthrax.osd.mil.

Information on Vaccine Safety

Do Vaccines Cause That?! A Guide for Evaluating Vaccine Safety Concerns, by Martin Myers, M.D., and Diego Pineda, M.S. (Galveston, TX: I4PH Press, 2008), discusses vaccination controversies and explains how to evaluate information you hear or read about vaccines.

The Johns Hopkins Bloomberg School of Public Health's Institute for Vaccine Safety lists recent scientific studies about vaccines, available at www.vaccinesafety.edu.

Information on Vaccines and Autism

Autism's False Prophets: Bad Science, Risky Medicine, and the Search for a Cure, by Paul A. Offit, M.D. (New York: Columbia University Press, 2008), explains the sources of the controversies surrounding autism; the measles, mumps, and rubella (MMR) vaccine; and the vaccine preservative thimerosal.

The nonprofit organization Autism Speaks raises awareness about autism and funds research to find new treatments for the disorder. You can find them at www.AutismSpeaks.org.

Resources

A variety of information is available free online to learn more about trials, insurance, regional requirements, injuries, and more.

Clinical Trial Resources

For information about clinical trials or to find a clinical trial for a specific disease, visit the National Institute of Health website, at www.clinicaltrials.gov.

To research or join a cancer clinical trial, visit the National Cancer Institute's website at www.cancer.gov/clinicaltrials.

To research and join an HIV/AIDS clinical trial, visit www.aidsinfo.nih.gov or call 1-800-874-2572.

Travel Resources

The CDC provides health and safety tips for travelers at www.cdc.gov/travel. You can also call the CDC for information about countries you plan to visit at 1-877-FYI-TRIP (1-877-394-8747).

The U.S. Department of State has travel tips and health information online at http://travel.state.gov/.

The CDC's Vessel Sanitation Program provides sanitation ratings for cruise ships at http://cdc.gov/nceh/vsp.

Travel medicine clinics can provide vaccinations and vaccination documentation needed to enter certain countries. These organizations can help you find a travel medicine clinic near you:

- The CDC at www.cdc.gov/travel (or call 1-800-232-4636)

- The International Society of Travel Medicine at www.istm.org (or call 770-736-7060)

- The American Society of Tropical Medicine and Hygiene at www.astmh.org (or call 847-480-9592)

To find a yellow fever vaccination clinic that can provide an International Certificate of Vaccination or Prophylaxis, visit www.cdc.gov/travel.

To stay updated on travel risks abroad, sign up for travelers' health e-mail updates at www.cdc.gov/emailupdates.

To learn about the health documentation required when you travel abroad, and to learn more about health insurance coverage for travelers, visit the U.S. Department of State's Medical Information for Americans Abroad web page at http://travel.state.gov/travel/tips/brochures/brochures_1215.html.

The CDC can answer your questions about international travel vaccinations at 1-877-394-8747.

The U.S. Embassy or Consulate in a host country can help you find medical care in an emergency. Find a country's embassy or consulate online at http://usembassy.state.gov.

Health Insurance Resources

Needy families can get free childhood vaccines through the Vaccines for Children program by calling the CDC at 1-800-232-4636 or by visiting www.cdc.gov/vaccines/programs/vfc/contacts-state.htm.

To find affordable health-care insurance for children, visit the U.S. Department of Health and Human Services website, www.insurekidsnow.gov, or call 1-877-543-7669. Information is available in English and Spanish.

State Resources

To learn what vaccinations are required for school entry in your state, visit the National Network for Immunization Information's website at www.immunizationinfo.org/VaccineInfo/index.cfm.

To find your state health department, visit the CDC's website at www.cdc.gov/mmwr/international/relres.html.

Vaccine Injuries and Side Effects

The Vaccine Adverse Events Reporting System (VAERS) reports are available at http://vaers.hhs.gov. To file a VAERS report, use a form from the VAERS website, http://vaers.hhs.gov/. You can submit the form online, fax it to 1-877-721-0366, or mail it to VAERS, PO Box 1100, Rockville, MD, 20849-1100. You can contact VAERS at 1-800-822-7967 or e-mail info@vaers.org.

To learn more about the National Vaccine Injury Compensation Program, visit www.hrsa.gov/vaccinecompensation/, or call 1-800-338-2382.

Learn about the potential side effects of each vaccine at the CDC's Possible Side-Effects from Vaccines web page at www.cdc.gov/vaccines/vac-gen/side-effects.htm.

Vaccination Quiz

The CDC's Interactive Adolescent and Adult Quiz can tell you the vaccines you might need. The quiz is located at http://www2.cdc.gov/nip/adultImmSched/.

Vaccine Shortages

The latest vaccine shortages are posted on the CDC website at www.cdc.gov/vaccines/vac-gen/shortages.

Common Acronyms for Vaccines and Vaccine-Preventable Diseases

BCG   Bacille Calmette-Guérand vaccine, a tuberculosis vaccine

DTaP   Diphtheria, tetanus, and acellular pertussis vaccine

DTP   Diphtheria, tetanus, and (whole-cell) pertussis vaccine

Hib   *Haemophilus influenzae* type b

HPV   Human papillomavirus

IPV   Inactivated polio vaccine

JE   Japanese encephalitis

LAIV   Live, attenuated influenza vaccine

MCV4   Meningococcal conjugate vaccine

MDR TB   Multidrug-resistant tuberculosis

MMR   Measles, mumps, and rubella

MMRV   Measles, mumps, rubella, and varicella

MPSV4   Meningococcal polysaccharide vaccine

OPV   Oral polio vaccine (live)

PCV or PCV7   Pneumococcal conjugate vaccine, used mostly on children

PPS, PPSV, PPV, or PPV23   Pneumococcal polysaccharide vaccine, used on children and adults

RV   Rotavirus

TB   Tuberculosis

Td   Tetanus and diphtheria vaccine

Tdap   Tetanus, diphtheria, and acellular pertussis booster

XDR TB   Extensively drug-resistant tuberculosis

YF   Yellow fever

Appendix D

Vaccine Records

Childhood Vaccine Record: Newborn to 18

Vaccine	Recommended Schedule (as of 2009)	Date of Vaccination	Notes
Hepatitis B	Birth		
	1–2 months		
	4 months (if using combination vaccine)		
	6–18 months		
Rotavirus	2 months		
	4 months		
	6 months (some brands)		
DTaP	2 months		
	4 months		
	6 months		
	15–18 months		
	4–6 years		
Hib	2 months		
	4 months		
	6 months (some brands)		
	12–15 months		
Pneumococcal	2 months		
	4 months		
	6 months		
	12–15 months		
Polio (IPV)	2 months		
	4 months		
	6–18 months		
	4–6 years		

Vaccine	Recommended Schedule (as of 2009)	Date of Vaccination	Notes
MMR *	12–15 months		
	4–6 years		
Varicella *	12–15 months		
	4–6 years		
Hepatitis A	12–18 months, dose 1; dose 2, at least 6 months after dose 1		
Meningococcal (MCV4)	11–12 years (can be younger for high-risk kids)		
Tdap	11–12 years (can be 10 years for one brand)		
HPV	11–12 years, dose 1 (can be as young as 9 years); dose 2, 2 months after dose 1; dose 3, at least 6 months after dose 1		

* The MMR and varicella vaccinations are not recommended for children with certain immune system problems, or if a young adult is pregnant.

Vaccine	Recommended Schedule (as of 2009)	Date of Vaccination	Notes
Influenza (LAIV only approved for ages 2 and up) *	6 months or older, dose 1		
	7 months or older, dose 2; at least 4 weeks after dose 1		
	Age 2		
	Age 3		
	Age 4		
	Age 5		
	Age 6		
	Age 7		
	Age 8		
	Age 9		
	Age 10		
	Age 11		
	Age 12		
	Age 13		
	Age 14		
	Age 15		
	Age 16		
	Age 17		
	Age 18		

* The LAIV vaccination is not recommended for children with certain immune system problems, or if a young adult is pregnant.

Adult Vaccine Record: Ages 19 and Older

Vaccine	Recommended Schedule (as of 2009)	Date of Vaccination	Notes
Tdap or Td	Every 10 years; one dose might be Tdap and the rest Td		
HPV	For women 26 and younger, dose 1; dose 2, 2 months after dose 1; dose 3, at least 6 months after dose 1		
Varicella *	Dose 1, if not already immune to chickenpox; dose 2, at least 4 weeks after dose 1		
Varicella Zoster (shingles) *	For adults 60 and older, 1 dose		
MMR *, for adults born on or after 1957 who are not immune	For adults born on or after 1957 who are not immune, 1 to 2 doses, depending on vaccination history, health, and circumstance		
Pneumococcal, if you are 65 or older	For adults 65 or older or who have certain illnesses, 1 dose		

The varicella, zoster, and MMR vaccinations are not recommended for those with certain immune system problems, or those who are pregnant.

Vaccine	Recommended Schedule (as of 2009)	Date of Vaccination	Notes
Influenza (Inactivated or LAIV) *	Yearly for adults 50 and over; also for younger adults depending on age, health, occupation, and circumstance		
	2010		
	2011		
	2012		
	2013		
	2014		
	2015		
	2016		
	2017		
	2018		
	2019		
	2020		

* The LAIV vaccination is not recommended for those with certain immune system problems, or those who are pregnant.

Other vaccinations might be necessary depending on health, lifestyle, occupation, race, travel plans, and other circumstances. Ask your health-care provider whether you need to be vaccinated against the following:

◆ Hepatitis A

◆ Hepatitis B

◆ Meningococcal disease (MCV4 or MPSV4)

◆ Hib

◆ Typhoid

◆ Polio (IPV)

- Yellow Fever
- Japanese encephalitis
- Rabies (prophylactic)
- Anthrax
- Smallpox
- Tuberculosis (BCG)

Other Vaccinations

Vaccination	Recommended Schedule	Date of Vaccination	Notes

Index

B

W-X-Y-Z

Check Out BEST-SELLERS

READ BY MILLIONS!

BOCA RATON PUBLIC LIBRARY, FLORIDA
3 3656 0512755 1

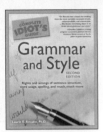

Grammar and Style SECOND EDITION
978-1-59257-115-4
$16.95

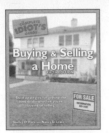

Buying & Selling a Home
978-1-59257-458-2
$19.95

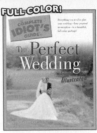

FULL COLOR!
The **Perfect Wedding** Illustrated
978-1-59257-566-4
$22.95

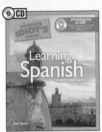

CD
Learning Spanish FOURTH EDITION
978-1-59257-485-8
$24.95

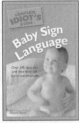

Baby Sign Language
978-1-59257-469-8
$14.95

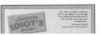

614.47 Smi
Smith, Michael Joseph.
The complete idiot's guide
to vaccinations

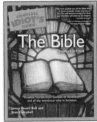

The Bible THIRD EDITION
978-1-59257-389-9
$18.95

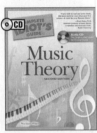

CD
Music Theory SECOND EDITION
978-1-59257-437-7
$19.95

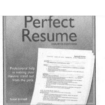

Perfect Resume FOURTH EDITION
978-1-59257-463-6
$14.95

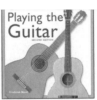

Playing the Guitar SECOND EDITION
978-0-02864244-4
$21.95

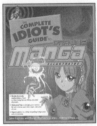

Manga
978-1-59257-335-6
$19.95

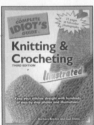

Knitting & Crocheting THIRD EDITION Illustrated
978-1-59257-491-9
$19.95

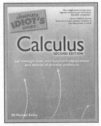

Calculus SECOND EDITION
978-1-59257-471-1
$18.95

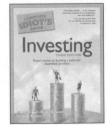

Investing THIRD EDITION
978-1-59257-480-3
$19.95

More than **450 titles** available at booksellers and online retailers everywhere

ALPHA

www.idiotsguides.com